Keto Diet For Beginners

How To Go On The Ketogenic Diet

Easy and Delicious Keto Recipes And An 8 Week Keto Meal Plan

Wing Horse Media Circles

Will Ramos

Table of Contents

Chapter 1:
Starting Your Keto Journey

The Ketogenic Diet – or Keto Diet for short – is powerful. It's life changing in every sense of the word. While weight loss is probably one of the reasons you picked up this book, it's just one of the unexpected and beautiful side effects of eating in a way that benefits your entire physical well being

What else can you expect when eating the Keto Diet way?

You'll regain your health. We'll go into this in much more detail throughout the following chapters, but suffice it to say, the way you're eating today – and the way you've largely been taught to eat in this American culture – is not healthy. You probably already have this belief yourself, as you're surrounded by fast food restaurants, fried food eateries, convenience stores that sell every non-healthy item, and even your own grocery store is to blame, stuffed with nutritionally deficient food products.

Yuck!

But after being on the Ketogenic Diet for one month – that's right, just four weeks – you'll see a remarkable difference in your health. You'll regain it and feel better overall – more energy, sleeping better, waking up refreshed, and weight loss, too.

What You'll Find Here

Inside this Ketogenic Diet book, you'll find all of the following and more:

- Dietary information backed up by real science, not bogus claims peddled by 'get rich quick' diet gurus
- A breakdown of why your body functions best in ketosis
- The exact Keto Diet success formula you'll follow
- Learning all about the ingredients you'll buy to stock your kitchen
- Not just one 4 week meal plan, but two – a basic plan and a 30-minute meal plan
- A complete and detailed step-by-step plan to get your body into ketosis
- Help and troubleshooting to mitigate potential side effects (none of which are harmful!)
- Dozens of helpful tips and tricks to fully integrate the Keto diet into not your neighbor's life – but yours!

Think of this book as the Ketogenic Diet all-in-one handy manual you've been looking for! We're not going to give you some vague advice, three recipes, and send you out into the confusing food landscape to fend for yourself. Nope, not at all! This book is here to guide you, help you, and encourage you every step of the way. There are big dietary changes in store for you, so come with us and enjoy the journey!

Trying Diet After Diet

The diet merry-go-round is confusing, dizzying, and doesn't get you anywhere. You just keep going in circles. Even if you do make a little bit of progress for a few weeks or months, it's not enough progress and doesn't motivate you.

That doesn't mean you are destined to fail at diets or will never be able to succeed on one.

It just means the diet is flawed!

It's hard to try another diet, because behind you in your past is a bunch of dieting mistakes that haven't worked. Diets are disappointing. You see the "before and after" pictures of people in magazines, on TV, and online, and you want that to be you.

A diet is just a meal plan. Right now, you're already on a diet. But it's not working. It's not bringing you the results that you want, it's not bringing you the body you want, and it's not bringing you any closer towards the future that you want.

So, let's try a new diet, one which will work. It will bring you closer to the results you want.

A Diet Based on Your Actual Body

What is this new diet? It's called the Ketogenic Diet, or Keto Diet for short. It's called the ketogenic diet because we'll be changing your body's natural metabolic processes from using unhelpful fuel to using helpful fuel (as well as stored fuel, too!)

Your body is amazing and needs lots of fuel every day to keep you mentally alert, keep your body systems functioning properly, to physically move you, and to do all the things you need to do throughout your life. Everything you eat becomes this fuel.

But some fuel is better than others. Some fuel (carbohydrates, sugars) is going to give you a quick burst of energy, and then the rest get stored. Other fuel (good fats, proteins) is going to not only give you better, more sustained and long-lasting energy, but will also start up a whole new metabolic process in your cells that burns the stored fuel. Pretty cool, huh?

We're not bashing carbs and sugars here, but they're just not sufficient enough for the complex and wonderful physical body you have. They're largely insufficient as a fuel source. It would be like trying to run a campfire on twigs. Sure, you get a little heat and light. But, wouldn't you want more substantial fuel, like thick logs? That's basically why the Ketogenic Diet switches up your fuel source from carbohydrates and sugars to fats and proteins. You can't run your body on twigs!

The Ketogenic Diet is designed to put your body into a metabolic state called *ketosis.* Ketosis is not a singular bodily function, but rather a series of processes that activate certain cells to stop doing things they were before and start doing new things. When your body goes into ketosis, it's kind of like having a change in an upper level position. New management comes in to switch policies around.

Your body is going to be using different energy sources than it was before.

Your Metabolism Process

So, ketosis is a metabolic state. But, what exactly does that mean?

When we're talking about your metabolism, we're actually talking about specifically how your body takes in energy from the foods you eat, processes it, and either stores it or uses it for fuel. Your metabolism takes this entire energy life cycle into account. When we say, "Oh, she has a high metabolism," we mean that the entire process of assimilating foods and using them for energy is functioning at its peak potential.

You can see the process listed out here:

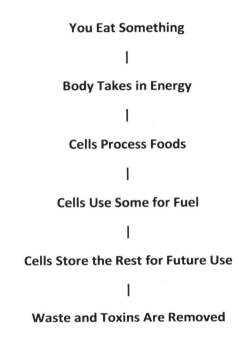

You Eat Something

|

Body Takes in Energy

|

Cells Process Foods

|

Cells Use Some for Fuel

|

Cells Store the Rest for Future Use

|

Waste and Toxins Are Removed

This cycle is continuously operating every day of your life. Every time you eat something, the nutrients in those foods enter the metabolic cycle and go through the whole process. Your body is like a metabolism factory, continuously processing incoming shipments. Those 'shipments' are the different chemical components of the foods that you eat: fats, proteins, carbohydrates, sugars, starches, fiber, vitamins, and minerals.

A Storage Solution That Works Against You

Many storage solutions are very helpful. But, unfortunately, the body's natural ability to store extra energy is working against you in the fight to lose weight.

If our bodies didn't have a built-in storage function, then none of us would ever need to lose weight! It wouldn't be stored in our cells in the first place. But, this was a survival mechanism from thousands of years ago, when obtaining foods year round was much more difficult than it is today. Your body developed 'storage spaces' for cells to deposit that unused energy to use it for a future time. Without out, Homo sapiens would surely have died out during the long, cold European winters. We absolutely needed that stored energy.

The problem today is, of course, our lifestyles have become so convenient, every single type of food is so plentiful, and we don't have enough natural exercise integrated into that lifestyle. We don't have a starvation winter period in our lives anymore. We just keep eating what we want every day. But, our body's metabolic process hasn't changed. It doesn't know that it's the 21st century. Your body still thinks it's 30,000 years ago and keeps storing and storing. That storage gets larger and larger, resulting in weight gain.

This is why it's so easy to gain weight in the 21st century. You have an ancient survival mechanism to fight against.

How do we change this process?

There is a way – and that's by changing your metabolic state to go into ketosis.

Ketosis utilizes that stored energy *in addition to* the energy that you're eating that day. It's burning the fat your body stored two weeks ago, two months ago, or even two years ago. Ketosis changes the metabolism cycle – and changes how your body uses that stored energy.

What is This Stored Energy?

The stored energy in your cells doesn't come from every single food you eat. It only comes from foods containing glucose, which is primarily found in carbohydrates. Glucose is a small sugar molecule.

That's right – carbohydrates become glucose, which becomes extra stored energy, isn't burned off by your normal daily body functions, and makes you gain weight.

The Carbohydrate Life Cycle

Let's look at the metabolic life cycle of a carbohydrate in your body.

Step 1:

You're at a birthday party and decide to eat a slice of cake. Hey, it's super yummy! Cake is made with white flour and sugar, both of which are carbohydrates. It also has eggs.

Step 2:

As soon as the cake enters your stomach, those nutrients are broken down. The protein and fat in the eggs is used as energy. The carbohydrates from the flour and sugar are turned into glucose.

Step 3:

You need more energy to have fun at the party, so a small amount of glucose is used as energy that day. But not all of it is needed. Plus, your body is specifically designed to store extra glucose. You might need that energy later.

Step 4:

The extra glucose is deposited into your cells for storage, causing you to gain weight from eating the cake.

Step 5:

The weight that you are trying to lose is still there. Your body didn't use it as energy at the party. Also, now you've added to the weight by eating more carbohydrates. There's also a huge chance you won't go through a 'starvation period' in the near future. You'll go back to step 1, eating more carbohydrates and only using the glucose as energy that day, never touching the stored fat you want to lose.

Yes, it's frustrating to be stuck in this type of carbohydrate metabolic cycle. It's happening every day when you eat bread, pasta, white flour goods, rice, and other whole grains. These carbohydrates have nowhere to go but right into the storage areas. They're not utilized by your cells. Also, your body isn't using the existing energy storage, either. It's just piling more and more glucose molecules into your cells. The number on the scale goes up, and not even a weekly exercise routine helps it go back down again.

That's why you need to switch your body from a carbohydrate metabolic state to a ketosis metabolic state.

So, What Exactly is Ketosis?

When your body is in ketosis, your liver is the organ that helps you out the most. It starts producing ketones that work in tandem with your energy storage cells to take that energy out of the cells and use it.

Ketones are a byproduct that's created when your body breaks down 'good fats' for energy while at the same time your carbohydrate intake (glucose intake) is low. We'll talk more about 'good fats' to eat later in this chapter.

When you stop eating carbohydrate heavy foods, you drastically reduce the amount of glucose entering your system. Your body is naturally wired to use glucose for fuel, right? So, when there isn't a lot of it coming in, your body has to look elsewhere for fuel.

In this case, it's fat – the stored energy in your cells.

So, your body goes to those fat storage cells and starts using those for energy. This process is called beta-oxidation because it uses oxygen atoms. After beta-oxidation is finished, what you get is a ketone. That ketone is then used as fuel for your daily energy. This whole new metabolic cycle is called ketosis.

Let's take a look at all the steps in this process:

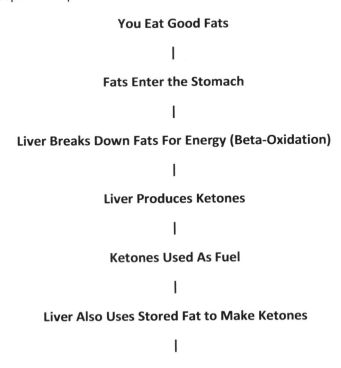

You Eat Good Fats

|

Fats Enter the Stomach

|

Liver Breaks Down Fats For Energy (Beta-Oxidation)

|

Liver Produces Ketones

|

Ketones Used As Fuel

|

Liver Also Uses Stored Fat to Make Ketones

|

The Ketogenic Diet reduces carbohydrates to such a tiny amount in your diet and raises your 'good fat' intake to such a high percentage of your diet, that it kicks your body into ketosis.

Ketosis is the metabolic state that helps you burn stored energy – and gain all those wonderful benefits.

My Ketogenic Story

There are so many hidden carbohydrates (including all kinds of sugars) lurking in the foods you eat, that even someone who appears healthy on the outside can suffer from unexpected and severe health problems on the inside.

That's exactly what happened to me. I was a hale and healthy male athlete in my teens! I was playing sports, getting outside a lot, didn't carry any extra weight, and my BMI was totally normal. If you saw me, you'd have no idea that I was secretly unhealthy. I sure didn't know.

So, imagine my total surprise when I was suddenly diagnosed with diabetes.

Wait, what?

Yeah, whatever stereotypes you think about the average diabetes sufferer, that surely wasn't me. But suddenly, it was. I now had a disease that radically changed my relationship with food. I'd always exercised frequently, that I just didn't think it was necessary or important to care about what was on the plate. I just burned all those calories, anyway.

But diabetes has nothing to do with calories, being thin, exercising, or sports. That was eye-opening. I was thrown for a loop and struggled with my life into my early adulthood, trying everything I could think of to lessen my symptoms and get my diabetes under control. It took longer than I want to admit (especially to you!) to finally realize there was this incredible link between diet and health. Hey, I was a teenager okay?

Yet, once I recognized this link, my whole outlook changed immediately. I started with the Atkins Diet, which was popular at the time, then shortly thereafter started exploring the Keto Diet. This was around the early 2000s. The Ketogenic Diet sounded weird and extreme to me, with its ridiculously high fat contents and ridiculously low carb contents, but hey – I was already experimenting, so why not?

Well, needless to say, that Keto Diet experiment turned into a full tilt obsession as soon as my diabetes numbers started looking healthier. The more I ate this diet, the better my numbers got. Each doctor visit I was improving. I read everything I could get my hands on, including all about the nutrition, the science, the practical application, the recipes, and the meal plans. I absorbed this knowledge even better than a sponge, because my own health was at stake!

My experiments and personal field tested knowledge paid off. You might not believe me, but it's the truth:

The diabetes is gone. A long gone memory by this point.

And, I've been on the Ketogenic Diet for fourteen years.

I changed the metabolic process in my own body, I'm in ketosis 100% of the time, and I've never been healthier. On the inside and the outside this time.

Your Future Story

Ten years from now, you're going to be telling a story about your health to someone. "Back ten years ago, I'd never been on the Ketogenic Diet, but I was struggling with my weight and health. As soon as I got on it, I felt better and have never looked back."

Let's make that your real story. Let's eat for your real body and what it needs every day of your life. Let's go Keto – and never look back!

Chapter 2:
Why You Want Get Into The Keto Lifestyle

Besides weight loss, there are many other benefits to being in a ketosis metabolic state on the Ketogenic Diet. They can be basically grouped into two categories:

- Health
- Lifestyle

We'll go into each one of these in detail, so that you get a complete understanding of how this diet can help you.

7 Benefits of Keto for Your Health

1. Keto for Diabetes

The sugar in your blood sugar is insulin, which also comes from carbohydrates. When you eat too many carbohydrates, then you also increase the amount of insulin in your blood stream. This creates a spike of energy, which you might think of as a 'sugar high.' But after every high comes a crash. Then you reach for more carbohydrates and sugars to spike again. This spike-crash-spike-crash cycle is bad for your health. Staying in ketosis stabilizes your blood sugar.

When you think 'blood sugar,' you've got to also think about your body's energy that's processed as part of your overall metabolism. Your blood moves along the interior highway of your artery and vein system, carrying nutrients from the food you eat to every part of your body.

However, just like a polluted river, blood can also become clogged with too much glucose. That glucose wasn't processed by your liver, so it ends up in your blood stream, elevating your blood sugar levels. The sugars and carbs you eat end up in your blood stream, spiking your energy levels.

You spike your blood sugar, you receive a spike of energy. That doesn't seem so bad. A quick burst of energy is good from time to time. But with every spike comes an opposite reaction of the crash. That crash is not healthy and represents too much of a change in your blood sugar. It also makes you feel sluggish, mentally foggy, drained, and it also interferes with your natural sleep cycle. As a result, in order to feel that burst of energy again, you're naturally going to – you guessed it – reach for something else to spike your blood sugar.

If you repeat this spike-crash-spike-crash cycle too often, you're sending your blood sugar on an unnecessary and unhealthy roller coaster that can have long-term negative consequences. However, if you go into the ketosis metabolic state, your blood sugar won't get stuck in this cycle, thus preventing and helping diabetes.

2. Keto for Metabolic Syndrome

The Ketogenic Diet helps those who struggle with metabolic syndrome and its problems: an expanded waistline, low HDL levels, and high blood pressure, triglyceride levels, and blood sugar. This diet will lower your insulin levels, stabilize your blood sugar, and reduces your blood pressure. It's ideal for metabolic syndrome.

3. Keto for Brain Health

It goes without saying that your brain is unbelievably important – and when your diet doesn't support brain health, you can feel it. You have problems with memory, nerve function, your vision, alertness, and struggle with brain fog. On the Keto Diet, your brain is fueled both by protein and ketones. Also, since your brain requires so much energy, your liver will start producing making new glucose in a process called gluconeogenesis. Your liver takes the glycerol from the fatty acids present in triglycerides, which are the fats your body stores, turns them into glucose, and sends them to the brain as fuel. In fact, the Keto Diet was first developed for those suffering with epilepsy – because it helps the brain so much.

4. Keto for Cancer

How can this new eating plan help cancer? Some initial research has linked the Keto Diet with slowing down the growth of tumors. Cell biologist Otto Warburg discovered cancer cells flourish due to their ability to ferment glucose. In other words, one of a cancer cell's primary food sources is – you guessed it – sugar. Eliminate the sugars and carbs from the diet, and the cancer cells become weakened and starved. More research in this area is required, but suffice it to say, it only makes sense that Keto helps reduce cancer.

5. Keto for Reduced Inflammation

When the body has difficulty healing itself and struggles to protect itself from illnesses, that's when you get inflammation. Inflammation has also proven to be the first symptom for many chronic conditions, including rheumatoid arthritis, atherosclerosis, periodontitis, hay fever, and even some cancers. But being on the Keto Diet reduces sugars derived from carbohydrates, which are a huge source of inflammation. Less sugar equals less inflammation.

6. Keto to Manage Cholesterol and Blood Pressure

Stabilizing your blood sugar helps give you a much better circulatory system, which in turn both manages and lowers cholesterol and helps your blood pressure. It's common knowledge to assume that heart problems come from eating too much fat, but that's not true. It's too many carbohydrates that cause problems. When you reduce carbs and eat good fats and proteins, you're giving your heart what it needs.

A lot of people also think more fat equals higher cholesterol, but your body knows how to maintain cholesterol homeostasis. Those sugars stay in your bloodstream, while the cholesterol you eat (in the good fats mentioned in the next chapter) attaches to lipoproteins and is transported to your cells and organs. HDL is this high density lipoprotein. In essence, you want to eat these good fats, which we'll explain more in the chapter on your Macros! That helps balance your cholesterol and increase the overall health of your entire circulatory system.

7. Keto for Fatty Liver Disease

As you've read in this book, your liver is the main organ switching you from a carbohydrate metabolic state to a ketosis state. It produces ketones. Your liver acts as a filter, helping to separate good nutrients from bad and send the bad nutrients to your kidneys to be flushed out. Fatty liver disease comes when you're consuming so many sugars and carbs (usually through alcohol), that your body isn't burning any stored fat and instead is depositing it on your liver. Once you stop consuming such high quantities of carbohydrates, your body will then start burning the fat deposits on your liver – and any other organ as well.

7 Benefits of Keto for Your Lifestyle

1. Natural Weight Loss

This is definitely the most obvious benefit, and not just because you're cutting out nearly an entire food group! When your body is in ketosis, it's designed to burn the extra fat stores in your cells. That contributes to a natural and healthy weight loss. Your weight loss amounts will vary depending on how much weight you have to lose and the percentage of fat in your body. But you will see a difference!

2. Hunger Management

When you eat carbs and sugars, you enter the blood sugar spike-crash-spike cycle mentioned above. That quick energy doesn't sustain your appetite at all, which you've probably noticed. Those simple carbohydrates and sugars are burned so quickly that you get hungry again in a short period of time. But when you replace those ingredients with the good fats and proteins, your hunger pangs will be greatly reduced. Instead of reaching for toast or pancakes in the morning, try an egg omelet with bacon and cheese. You'll feel full for hours! We give plenty of breakfast options here to stave off hunger at any time of the day!

3. Better Appetite Control

You've probably tried diets in the past that left you constantly hungry. Low fat meals and simple carbohydrates like bread, biscuits, fruit, or cookies not only don't satisfy your hunger, they actually make you more hungry in the long run! That's why humans are more apt to develop sugar cravings rather than meat cravings. Calm your cravings down and help bring your appetite under control by following the Keto Diet. It's an unexpected and amazing benefit!

4. More Energy

Your body was not just built to store fat, but to use the 'good fats' effectively as fuel. This helps to give you much more energy. It won't be the spike-crash style of sugary laden energy, either. You will have plentiful, sustained energy that keeps you going all day and won't make you feel exhausted in the afternoon. The Keto Diet is built for a high performance lifestyle. This is also shown in nature, too; carnivores have to expend more energy than herbivores just to catch their prey, so they rely on a high fat, high protein diet. Humans are omnivores, but our brain and muscles require incredible amounts of calories for daily use. Switch those calories to the perfect Macro percentage, and you'll get more energy than you ever dreamed of.

You'll also avoid what's commonly nicknamed the 'carb coma,' which happens when you feel sleepy after consuming too many carbohydrates!

5. Mental Clarity

Your brain requires hundreds of calories per day to process all of its intricate functions. Not to mention when you decide to learn something new, take a class, speak a foreign language, or just need that gray matter to get through a stressful day at the office. When you eat 'good fats' and proteins, those nutrients give your mind the power it needs.

Thus, you not only feel more mentally alert, but everything associated with your brain is increased. You'll remember things better, you'll have an easier time coming up with new ideas, you'll retain more information, and overall, you'll learn better. This is especially important if you work in a field that requires heavy brainpower, like marketing, the arts, and other creative professions.

6. Burn Fat for Fuel

This benefit is the heart of what makes being in a ketosis metabolic state so incredible. Your cells aren't using just the fuel you're eating now; they're also using the stored fuel. When your body uses stored fat from your cells for fuel, that fat disappears off your body, thus decreasing your weight. That fat is gone – because it was used! Think of the Ketogenic Diet as a fat decluttering nutrition plan. You're cleaning out your cells of fat that's been stored there for a long time, perhaps even years. The longer you're in ketosis, the more frequently this process occurs. It's a win-win situation.

7. Better Mood and Emotions

If you've struggled with mood swings and emotions that frequently vacillate, then you'll find the Ketogenic Diet to be a breath of fresh air. You'll get out of the blood sugar spike-crash-spike cycle and you'll stabilize your emotions as well. Your brain will use protein and the ketones from your liver as fuel, which is excellent for the neurotransmitters in your brain to produce the 'good' hormones like serotonin, dopamine, and endorphins. That alone will do wonders for your mood and is a great, unexpected, and useful benefit

Is the Keto Diet for Everyone?

While being in ketosis is a metabolic state any human body can achieve, not everyone should be on the Keto Diet. As a disclaimer, we want to advise you to consult a doctor or certified nutritionist before beginning this diet. There are rare conditions like Muscular Dystrophy and conditions that affect certain organs like your kidneys, liver, or pancreas. Also, if you have a digestive disorder affecting your blood sugar, such as hypoglycemia or Type 1 diabetes. Yes, ketosis helped my diabetes, but I also want to caution you. As for Type 2 diabetes, I also advise you to consult a physician.

The Keto Diet is not recommended if you're pregnant, have gestational diabetes, or are nursing. Everything you eat affects your baby, so please don't change your diet until after your baby's been weaned. Suffering from an eating disorder wreaks havoc with both your mind and body, so don't attempt this diet at that time.

Once you've been cleared, then you're good to proceed!

Confusion Leads to Bad Press About Ketosis

You might have heard or read some bad press about the Keto Diet. It's jumped in popularity and has attracted its fair share of naysayers. They say that the diet is unhealthy, gives you weight gain rather than weight loss, messes with your blood sugar, leads to long term liver problems, and other negative claims.

Ketosis is NOT Ketoacidosis – Here's the Difference!

Most of this confusion comes from differentiating between two similar sounding conditions: ketosis and ketoacidosis. Ketosis is the metabolic state whereby your liver is producing ketones. By itself, it isn't harmful to your body at all. It just means you have a higher amount of ketones present in your blood and urine. But it isn't high enough to tip over into acidosis.

In fact, ketosis developed in our bodies thousands of years ago in human evolution as a way to use stored body energy during the winter, when fresh grains, sugars, and carbohydrates weren't plentiful. So, ketosis kept many of our ancestors alive in cold winters.

Ketoacidosis is completely different and yes, it is harmful. It's known as Diabetic Ketoacidosis (DKA). When your ketones are in dangerously high levels and your blood sugar is also too high, that makes your blood too acidic. When that happens, you have to seek medical attention immediately. But this condition usually only happens to those who not just have Type 1 or Type 2 diabetes, but whose bodies didn't produce any insulin or very poor amounts. If you produce insulin, then you're not in danger of your body developing DKA.

Symptoms of DKA include dehydration with extreme thirst and needing to urinate frequently, nausea, vomiting, stomach pain, low energy, and being short of breath. You'll be measuring your ketones using a breath meter or strips, so you'll know on a regular basis that you're in the good range.

So, ketosis is one of your body's natural functions (as a way to keep you alive during times of less food) and diabetic ketoacidosis is very harmful. They're very different!

What's the Keto Flu?

You'll find more in depth information about what's nicknamed the "Keto Flu" in Chapter 6, but briefly, this is the combination of flu-like symptoms you'll experience within the first 1-3 weeks of starting the Ketogenic Diet. Your body is adjusting to a completely new way of functioning, and it's a transition period.

These symptoms include:

- Low energy and fatigue
- Being brain foggy
- Headaches
- Being irritable and unmotivated
- Muscle cramps
- Nausea
- Sugar cravings (please don't give in!)

Luckily, these don't last too long and can be helped by drinking water with lemon to restore your electrolytes.

Now that you've read all about the benefits to being on the Keto Diet and how it's not harmful for your body, we're going to go into the practical advice. Read on to the next chapter to see what foods you can – and cannot eat!

Chapter 3:
Keto Foods: The Good And Bad

This chapter is when the rubber meets the road, and you'll find out exactly what you can – and can't – eat. We'll go food group by food group, navigating the confusing modern American landscape of food options from grocery stores to restaurants.

The Ketogenic Diet begins at the grocery store, and that's where you'll find the vast majority of ingredients to make recipes and meal plans.

But, before we send you off to stock up your cart, you need to be educated about what you're reading on food packages to find the best options.

Decoding Nutritional Labels

Food package nutritional labels give you all the information you need to say yes to Keto foods. Don't be blissfully unaware of the chemicals, additives, preservatives, and other food product 'bad guys' manufacturers shove into that brightly colored package. Yes, it looks enticing. But those aren't Keto Diet friendly food items. Study nutritional labels to really become familiar with what's exactly in the package. If you see carbs or sugars, put it back on the shelf.

Here are some red flag words to avoid:

- High Fructose Corn Syrup - It's nothing but sugar. Stay away!
- Enriched Flour / Wheat Flour / Corn Flour / Oat Flour - Carbs, carbs, and more carbs. Avoid anything with the word 'flour' in it.
- Partially Hydrogenated Oil – Stick to olive oil or coconut oil instead.
- Dextrose / Sucralose / Fructose / Lactose / Maltose – Anything with the suffix "ose" means sugar.
- Wheat Starch / Cornstarch – Starches are carbs.
- Aspartame / Saccharin / Acesulfame Potassium – Just fancy words for chemical sugars. Buy Stevia or anything with zero sugar.
- Lactitol / Sorbitol / Mannitol / Xylitol / Ethanol – More fancy words for sugar. These are sugar alcohols.
- Syrup – Liquid sugar. Yuck!

Food companies are pretty sneaky with the above ingredients. They'll stick them in supposedly harmless things like ketchup, barbecue sauce, ranch dressing, yogurt, and cheese. Get to know the red flag words, and you'll have a better chance on the Keto Diet.

Foods to Avoid

We thought we'd get the 'naughty list' out of the way first, so that you're aware of what you can't put in your grocery cart any longer. While this list is comprehensive, the foods you can eat is even more so!

Grains and Flours

Yes, this is the big "no no" category. Grain foods contain the highest amount of carbohydrates out of all the nutrition categories. Even if the product is gluten free, it's still not allowed on the Keto Diet.

Avoid:

- Bread
- Buns and rolls
- Bagels
- Biscuits
- Pasta and noodles
- Crackers of any flavor or shape
- Flour baked goods, like cakes, cookies, brownies, and pastries
- Pie crusts
- Pizza dough
- Donuts
- White flour and corn tortillas
- Cereals
- Rice
- Oats and oatmeal
- Other grains – barley, couscous, pilaf, pita, quinoa, etc.

Dairy

You get plenty of dairy options on the Ketogenic Diet, including an entire cheese selection. But there are a few dairy items you shouldn't have.

Avoid:

- Margarine in any form
- Cow's milk
- Sweetened milks
- Soymilk
- Evaporated milk
- Non-homemade whipped cream
- Ice cream
- Low-fat dairy items

Vegetables

We debunk the myth in this Ketogenic Diet book that all vegetables help you lose weight. But it is a pervasive myth, which is why we included our special veggie selection. Stick to those recommendations only. Otherwise, you'll be eating vegetables that are too high in carbs. Like these ones.

Avoid:

- Potatoes
- Sweet potatoes / yams
- Corn
- Carrots
- Leeks
- Peas
- Soybeans
- Beans – kidney beans, cannellini beans, black beans, etc.
- Any foods based on these vegetables, like refried beans, mashed potatoes, and French fries
- Any oils based on these vegetables, like corn oil and soybean oil

Fruits

Fruits are the second highest carbohydrate heavy foods. They just have way too much sugar. Think of fruits as colorful, sweet-smelling enemies that will subtly sabotage your diet!

Avoid:

- Apples
- Bananas
- Citrus – oranges, grapefruit, tangerines
- Melons – watermelon, honeydew, cantaloupe
- Grapes
- Pineapple
- Peaches
- All other fresh fruits – kiwi, papaya, mangoes, plums, etc.
- Fruit products – dried fruit, fruit juice, fruit popsicles, fruit candy, etc.

Packaged Meals

Packaged meals are some of the sneakiest items in the grocery store. They are often splashed with giant headlines like "all natural," "nutritious," and "complete meal." They're usually packed with carbs, sugars, and ridiculously high amounts of sodium.

Avoid:

- Canned soups
- Canned meals (Chef Boyardee, etc.)
- Boxed meal kits
- Frozen boxed meals
- Frozen breakfast sandwiches or wraps
- Frozen pizza
- Kids' lunch packaged meals
- Grocery store packaged foods or complete meals
- Pre-packaged sauce mixes
- Dried soup mixes

Snacks

Food manufacturers are incredibly good at getting you to buy their products by making them colorful, crunchy, and completely addicting. Some of these snacks say they're organic, all natural, healthy, or other bogus claims. Bypass them all. They'll not only stop your weight loss, they'll reverse it.

Avoid:

- Potato chips of any flavor
- Cheesy crunchy snacks (Cheetos, Cheese puffs, etc.)
- Pretzels
- Popcorn
- Tortilla chips
- Doritos of any flavor
- Rice cakes
- Cheese crackers, like Cheez-its and Goldfish
- Air popped crunchy snacks
- Any other packaged salty or cheesy snack food

Sweets

Sweet foods contain massive amounts of sugar, which will knock your body out of ketosis. Yeah, you don't want to do that. Although it seems counter-intuitive since many sweets are fat free, they are actually fattening to you. Please don't put these sugary sweets in your grocery cart.

Avoid:

- Candy
- Ice cream
- Frozen ice cream treats

- Popsicles
- Gum
- Canned cake frosting
- Plain white sugar
- Brown sugar
- Milk chocolate with a high sugar content
- Honey
- Any sweetener besides Stevia

Beverages

Americans love drinking our calories! Whether it's a grande latte in Starbucks, a soda at the movie theater, or an energy drink to help you through class, beverages are packed with sugars. Most of them are definitely on the avoid list.

Avoid:

- Soda, even if it says zero calories
- Energy drinks
- Sports drinks
- Coffee drinks
- Fruit juices
- Bottled or canned iced tea
- Alcohol, unless it's the occasional glass of approved wine

Foods You Can Eat!

So, we got the bad news out of the way with the foods you can't eat, but you have plenty of other options! We'll go through each of the major food groups and tell you exactly which foods you can have. If you were thinking that many Keto Diet ingredients are expensive and hard to find, then think again. You'll be purchasing produce, meats, dairy, herbs / spices, and some condiments. Find most of these are in your neighborhood grocery store. Some specialty ingredients might be found in a health food store or ordered online.

Beverages

Almond Milk - Regular cow's milk is not recommended on the Keto Diet, but you can definitely have almond milk. It comes in different flavors, like plain and vanilla. Be sure to get it unsweetened!

Coffee - Sheesh, a diet without coffee? Not the Keto Diet! Coffee by itself has an extremely low carb count, so you're safe to have your morning cup. Add a pinch of Stevia to sweeten it and pour on the heavy cream.

Tea - You might want to stock up your tea selection with a nice variety – black teas, green teas, herbal teas, and chai teas. A cup of English tea in the afternoon with a slice of lemon or a splash of heavy cream is a great pick-me-up.

Water – Make sure you're getting plenty of water on your Keto Diet. It helps flush out toxins, and your whole body needs it. You can have it with lemon or lime slices for some flavor and electrolytes.

Wine - Yes, you can have a little bit of wine on the Keto Diet. On average, wines have between 3 and 4 grams of carbohydrates per serving. White wines have less than red wines. Stick with Pinot Noir as a dry red and Pinot Blanc as a dry white. A small glass once or twice a week, as long as you factor in the carbs as part of your diet, can help you not feel deprived. You can use wine in cooking, too.

Meat, Fish & Eggs

Chicken – Chicken is such a huge source of both protein and fat that it must be included on here. Chicken also, well, tastes like chicken, so it takes to marinades and slow roasts really well.

Bacon – I know what you're thinking. A diet that helps me lose weight has *bacon* in it? Yes! In fact, bacon (look for nitrate-free and high quality bacon) is encouraged. Bacon has a magical mixture of both high fats and protein to give you the energy you need in the morning.

Beef – Yes, you can make Keto Diet burgers! Don't forget chili, too. Get some ground beef, roast beef, pot roast, sirloin tips, and steaks to cook and serve on the Keto Diet.

Eggs – One whole egg has 6 grams of protein and plenty of the good fats, so have fun eating eggs. They're a lot lower in protein than beef, pork, or chicken.

Fish – There are plenty of fish options on the Keto Diet, including cod, haddock, halibut, salmon, sea bass, trout, ahi tuna, and tilapia. Whatever kind of fish you purchase, make sure it is certified wild caught and hasn't been coated in carb heavy breading or fried.

Ham – You can get some ham to dice up for omelets and soups. Ham also makes a wonderful pairing with different cheeses. Make sure you're not getting ham with any sugar or honey curing.

Hot Dogs – Yep, good old fashioned beef franks are allowed on the Ketogenic Diet! Splurge on an all natural brand with the fewest fillers and the most fat.

Lamb – Ground lamb can be used as an alternative to ground pork or ground beef or ground turkey in a regular recipe to switch up your flavors! You can also purchase lamb chops and lamb tenderloin.

Meat Broth/Bouillon – Vegetable broth has too many carbs, so for making Keto soups, buy chicken broth and beef broth. Check the nutritional labels on chicken, beef, or fish bouillon cubes for their carb count. Some of them are made with wheat or whey powder.

Pork – Pork is delicious and carb free. There are many ways you can purchase it, including ground pork, pork shoulder, and pork tenderloin. You can also have pork rinds.

Prosciutto – Two slices of this popular Italian ham have 3 grams of fat.

Sausage – Store bought sausage often is stuffed with not just meat, but carb fillers. There's a recipe here in this book to make your own, which is a lot easier than you think!

Shrimp – Shrimp is a staple protein on the Ketogenic Diet, so stock up on either fresh or frozen. Homemade, unsweetened cocktail sauce goes very well with shrimp as a low carb appetizer.

Seafood – Besides fresh or frozen plain shrimp, you can also purchase many other types of seafood: scallops, crabs, mussels, clams, and even lobster. None of them have any carbs and make yummy dinner entrees.

Turkey – Turkey is not as high in fat as other forms of protein, so eat the dark meat only. One serving of roast dark meat has 5 grams of fat. You can also buy ground turkey.

Dairy

Brie – If you've never had this luscious, creamy cheese before, you're in for a tummy-pleasing treat. Definitely add it to your grocery cart.

Butter - For all of you butter lovers out there, this is the diet to be on! The Keto Diet encourages you to eat 70% of your calories from fat, and there is no fat tastier than butter. Buy unsalted, good quality butter in sticks or fresh from a farm.

Cheddar Cheese – One of the most popular cheeses in the world, you can purchase any style you like, except for a low fat version of course!

Colby Jack Cheese – A mild orange and white cheese that can be used in hundreds of recipes or eaten plain as a snack.

Cottage Cheese – Skip the low-fat version and go for the full fat instead, plain and with no fruit or flavorings added.

Cream Cheese – You want the full fat cream cheese, either in tubs or in blocks. None of that low-fat diet stuff from Philadelphia!

Feta Cheese – A creamy, yummy Mediterranean cheese for salads or to cook with.

Ghee – Ghee is Indian clarified butter, concentrating both the flavor and the fat. Each tablespoon has a whopping 12.7 grams of fat.

Goat Cheese – A unique tangy flavor makes goat cheese a great addition to Keto salads or as a snack. A 1 ounce serving has 8 grams of fat.

Greek Yogurt – Unsweetened and plain Greek yogurt is a yummy addition to the Keto Diet. It also provides probiotics to help balance good bacteria in your digestive tract.

Gruyere – Originally from Switzerland, this European cheese has 9 grams of fat per slice.

Heavy Cream – Say goodbye to low fat diets and hello to heavy cream. It has 12 grams of fat and no carbs, so add it to your tea, coffee, baked egg dishes, and soups.

Monterey Jack Cheese – This semi-hard cheese changes up regular flavors and is great with Mexican cuisine. It's filled with good fat, too.

Mozzarella Cheese – Even without pasta or garlic bread, you can still enjoy Italian food by having mozzarella cheese. Stringy and gooey, it's delicious.

Parmesan Cheese – A sprinkle of Parmesan brings wonderful Mediterranean flavor. Buy the full fat kind.

Sour Cream – With its light tang and creamy texture, sour cream is delicious in sauces, as a soup topping, and mixed with herbs for a dip.

Swiss Cheese – Holey Swiss cheese, Batman. You get 8 grams of fat per slice in this popular, tart cheese.

Vegetables

Arugula – This peppery tasting lettuce has 2.05 grams of carbohydrates and is a great base for Keto Diet friendly salads.

Asparagus – Only 1.78 grams of carbohydrates are in these fresh, crunchy vegetables. They're delicious when grilled, roasted, or wrapped in bacon.

Bell Pepper (Green) – The green bell peppers have less carbs than red, orange, or yellow, so buy that color only. They have 2.9 grams of carbs.

Bok Choy – This excellent Chinese vegetable is delicious in Asian soups or stir fries. Its carbohydrate count is only 1.18 grams. You can find it at Asian stores.

Broccoli – With 4 grams of carbs per cup, these little tree shaped veggies are a staple in the Keto kitchen. Buy them fresh or frozen.

Cabbage – With only 3 grams of carbohydrates, you can have cabbage on the Keto Diet. Only buy the green, since the red is much higher.

Cauliflower – You can chop up cauliflower, add cheese to it, or put it in stir fries. It has 2.9 carb grams per cup.

Chili Peppers – There are quite a few that are Keto diet friendly, including the small Thai red chilis, ghost peppers, and jalapenos. One cup of sliced jalapenos has 6 grams of carbs.

Celery – With 1.37 grams of carbs per stalk, this is one of the best Keto Diet friendly vegetables. That's great news, since it's such a delicious snack food.

Cucumber – Made of 96 percent water and 1.9 grams of carbohydrates, cucumbers are one of the healthiest and most refreshing veggies.

Dark Greens – Dark leafy greens like Swiss chard, mustard greens, and turnip greens each have less than 5 grams of carbohydrates per serving, making them both healthy and ideal for the Keto Diet.

Eggplant – Eggplant is a delicious Mediterranean vegetable and has a low carb count, at only 2.88 grams.

Green Beans – There are 7 grams of carbohydrates per 1 cup of 1/2" cut pieces of this sweet, popular legume. Get them frozen, since they still have plenty of nutritional value.

Iceberg Lettuce – There isn't much nutritional value to iceberg lettuce, but at only 0.2 carbs per serving, you can't go wrong adding chopped leaves to salads or as burger toppings.

Kohlrabi – This funny looking vegetable is super Keto friendly and has 2.6 grams of carbs. Chop it up with cabbage and iceberg lettuce to make a slaw.

Mushrooms – Regular white button mushrooms have only 2.26 grams of carbs, so you're welcome to eat them! They are great marinated in olive oil, stuffed with cheeses, or as a Keto pizza topping.

Onions – Although onions have 7.64 grams of carbohydrates, making them a bit high, they're an essential ingredient in cooking. Green onions have 1.1 grams and shallots have 1.7 grams, so use those whenever you can.

Romaine Lettuce – Pick up some Romaine for Keto salads, topping on burgers, and to make lettuce wraps. Romaine has 2.8 grams of carbs per serving.

Spinach – Fresh or frozen, delicious spinach is Ketogenic Diet approved, with only 1.43 grams of carbohydrates. Mix it with other dark greens and arugula for a base to salads.

Tomatoes – Yes, tomatoes are great on this diet. They have 2.69 grams of carbohydrates per serving. They're actually a fruit, but are way lower in carbs than most fruits.

Turnips – While a bit high at 4.63 grams of carbohydrates, turnips are still low enough to be enjoyed as an autumn treat. They're delicious roasted or mashed.

Zucchini – Yummy zucchini has 2.11 grams of carbs and can be mixed with herbs and spices for a quick roast or made into 'noodles' (zoodles) for veggie pasta.

Fruits

Avocado – Although it's green and looks like a vegetable, avocados are technically a fruit. They only have 1.84 grams of carbohydrates and are very high in good fats. You can slice them over salads or make your own guacamole.

Blackberries – The fruit with the lowest net carbs, at 4.3 grams per ¾ cup. Please be diligent when consuming these berries, since those carbs add up quickly.

Lemon – Lemons have a bit higher carb count since they are fruits, but a squeeze of fresh lemon juice here or there only adds a few grams.

Lime – One lime has 7 grams of carbs, so you can have a small occasional splash of lime juice to flavor Mexican dishes.

Raspberries – No fruit is no-carb, but raspberries are a delicious treat. One cup contains 15 grams of carbs, so factor those into your Macros.
Strawberries – A world without strawberries would be a sad one, indeed. Each cup contains 11 grams of carbohydrates, but the flavor is worth it!

Herbs & Spices

Basil – One tablespoon of fresh basil has 0.1 grams of carbs. The dried version has more carbs, but it is still worth purchasing to create Italian flavored dishes.

Bay Leaves – No carbs in bay leaves! Keto soups taste so good with these flavored herbs. Don't forget to take them out of the soup before serving.

Black Pepper – Black pepper has no carbohydrates. Pair it with the sea salt below to spice up foods.

Cajun Spices – Pick up a canister of no carb Cajun spices to dress up salmon, shrimp, beef, or chicken.

Chili Powder – Make chili, Mexican dishes, and other meat marinades with low carb chili powder, at 1.6 grams per teaspoon.

Cilantro – This peppery tangy herb has less than 1 gram of carbs per Tablespoon of fresh leaves. Make your own salsa with cilantro, tomatoes, and onions.

Cinnamon – Warm and comforting, cinnamon is also low carb and great for the Keto diet.

Cumin – There are no carbs in ground cumin! This incredible spice is essential in many Southwestern, Mexican, and Indian dishes.

Curry Powder – Curry powder has a wonderful yellow color and exotic flavor. Each teaspoon has 1.16 grams of carbs.

Garlic – Each fresh garlic clove has 1 gram of carbs, which is much less than garlic powder or salt. Garlic is an essential cooking ingredient, so stock your kitchen with fresh heads of garlic.

Lemon Pepper – There are no carbs in this popular spice blend. It's delicious on chicken.

Oregano – Together with basil, oregano is a popular and low carb Italian herb, at less than 1 gram per teaspoon.

Parsley – Dried parsley has no carbs! It's great to sprinkle over meats and add to soups.

Rosemary – A delicious herb when paired with beef, rosemary has no carbs!

Sage – Sage doesn't have any carbohydrates, either, so use as much as you want in your cooking.

Sea Salt – Don't buy the regular table salt, since that's not no-carb like sea salt. You can purchase different sea salt flake sizes and varieties like Himalayan pink sea salt.

Tarragon – Ground tarragon is usually found in a popular herb blend called Herbs de Provence, which also has marjoram, thyme, and parsley. It has less than 1 gram of carbohydrates per teaspoon.

Thyme – Both fresh and ground thyme are also low carb, with less than 1 gram per teaspoon.

Nuts and Seeds

Almonds - Almonds have a fairly low carb count and are one of the most versatile nuts. They're also delicious for snacking, too.

Chia Seeds – Chia seeds are slightly high in carbohydrates, featuring 12 grams per ounce, but they also have 9 grams of fat. You'll find recipes for them in this book.

Hemp Seeds – Two tablespoons adds 6 grams of good fats to your smoothies and other recipes.

Macadamia Nuts - Have you ever tried these nuts before? They are now going to be one of your staple snacks, since they're not only very low in carbs, they're also really high in Omega 3 essential fatty acids.

Nut Butters - Peanut butter is a bit high in carbs, but it is also high in fat, so that makes it less likely to spike your blood sugar glucose levels. Try other nut butters like almond butter and macadamia nut butter. If you've plateaued on your weight loss or are stalling, then keep nut butters to a bare minimum or cut them out completely. They do contain higher carbs than other snacks.

Pecans - Pecans are very good in a nutty snack mix, in baking, or by themselves by the handful. A 1 ounce serving contains 20.4 grams of fat.

Pumpkin Seeds – Full of good fats, pumpkin seeds are salty and crunchy. A 1 ounce serving has 5 grams of fat.

Sesame Seeds – You get 4.5 grams of fat in each Tablespoon of these tiny, crunchy seeds. They make an excellent salad topping and are perfect in Asian cooking.

Sunflower Seeds – Packed with 14 grams of fat per ounce, you'll want to snack on toasted or roasted sunflower seeds. Mix them with other nuts and seeds for a delicious Keto friendly trail mix.

Tahini - Tahini, or sesame seed butter, is a great snack with celery sticks. It provides plenty of the daily fats you need on the Keto Diet, while also being extremely low carb.

Walnuts - Whether sprinkled over a salad, folded into batter for baking, added to other nuts and seeds for a mix, or eaten alone, walnuts are delicious. Just 1 ounce has 28 grams of fat.

Oils, Vinegars, and Condiments

Apple Cider Vinegar - Since apple cider vinegar is high in acetic acid, that helps reduce the glycemic response of carbohydrates. It contains enzymes that enhance your metabolizing of proteins and fats. It's an excellent vinegar.

Barbecue Sauce – Made from either a ketchup or mustard base and loaded with spices, many barbecue sauces are Keto Diet friendly. Buy ones that have no sugar or carbs added.

Coconut Milk – Each 13.5 ounce can of full fat coconut milk has 2 grams of carbohydrates, so stock up your pantry. Canned coconut milk is dairy free and very creamy, making it perfect for Thai or Indian curries, soups, and sauces.

Coconut Oil - You want some cold-pressed coconut oil. Coconut oil is one of the most useful things you can have in the house. It also is an essential ingredient in Keto Fat Bombs.

Curry Paste – You can find jars of pre-made Thai curry pastes (yellow, red, green) in the Asian section of your grocery store or at an Asian food market. These pastes are made up of distinctly strong herbs and spices that form a base for making amazing curries. They have between 1 and 3 grams of carbs per Tablespoon, depending on the brand.

Dill Pickles - Pickles are part of the fermented food group, along with sauerkraut. Pickles have natural acids that stabilize your blood sugar. Go for dill pickles that aren't as sweet as other kinds.

Fish Sauce – Thai and Vietnamese dishes use fish sauce, which is extremely low carb, at less than 1 gram per Tablespoon. It's so strongly flavored, which you can smell as soon as you open the bottle, that you don't need much. Use fish sauce in Asian soups and curries.

Flavored Oils – Flavored oils can become marinades for meat or fish, cooking oils, or homemade salad dressings. You can add many flavors to your pantry, including garlic oil, chili oil, rosemary oil, oregano oil, thyme oil, and basil oil. Choose the ones with the highest fat contents. They have no carbs!

Horseradish Sauce – Its distinct flavor and very low carb count make horseradish sauce a great condiment. There are 1.7 grams of carbohydrates per Tablespoon.

Ketchup – If you can find a natural ketchup made without sugar or high fructose corn syrup, then add it to your Ketogenic Diet pantry. Ketchup is a bit higher in carbs than mustard or mayo, because it's made with tomatoes. Use sparingly as a treat.

Lemon Juice / Lime Juice – Bottled lemon and lime juice can also be stocked in your pantry. A little goes a long way with these citrusy, tangy juices. They have higher carb counts than other condiments, so use sparingly.

Mayonnaise – Did you know that regular full fat (not diet) mayo has 0.5 grams of carbohydrates? It's a very Keto Diet friendly condiment. You can make both egg and chicken salads with mayo.

Mustard – Both classic yellow mustard and high quality Dijon mustard are excellent condiments for a low carb pantry. They hardly have any carbohydrates and no sugar, either. Use on chicken, beef, or pork dishes.

Olive Oil – Regular full fat olive oil is going to be one of your best sources of the good fats in the Keto Diet. You can pan fry chicken, drizzle it over salads, or even make homemade beauty products with it. Check nutritional labels to purchase the olive oils with the highest fat content in grams.

Pesto – Pesto is made with basil, garlic, pine nuts, and sometimes a splash of lemon juice. It's a delicious combination that gives you Italian flavor for chicken or beef dishes.

Ranch Dressing – Its creamy texture comes from dairy products and not carbs, so ranch dressing is okay to have on the Keto Diet. Choose a brand with the lowest sugar content you can find.

Red Wine Vinegar – Balsamic vinegar has too many carbs for the Keto diet, so substitute red wine vinegar instead. You can mix it with flavored oils to create your own salad dressings.

Soy Sauce – Asian cuisine wouldn't be the same without salty, delicious soy sauce. It's a low carb condiment that you can use as a flavoring in soups or as a marinade for beef, chicken, pork, or shrimp. There's about 1 gram of carbohydrates per Tablespoon.

Sriracha – This popular red Asian hot sauce is also low carb, at 1 gram per teaspoon. Find a brand that is completely sugar free. Drizzle it over salads, eggs, meats, or fish.

Tabasco – Another popular hot sauce, Tabasco has no carbs!

Tamari – This is another kind of soy sauce and is both gluten free and carbohydrate free. Get the reduced sodium kind to cut out more salt.

Tartar Sauce – You can make your own tartar sauce with mayonnaise and diced dill pickles, or you can purchase it premade. If you do get it bottled, read the labels and buy the brand with no sugar or carbs. It's delicious on fish!

Tomato Sauce – Buy plain, unsweetened tomato sauce and diced tomatoes in cans or jars. You'll also want some tomato paste, too. Although tomato is a fruit, it's very low in carbohydrates.

White Vinegar – You can not only cook with white vinegar, you can clean with it, too! It has no carbs and is an essential ingredient if you want to pickle onions or cucumbers.

White Wine Vinegar – Not to be confused with white vinegar, you can definitely have white wine vinegar on the Keto Diet. Its carb count is less than 1 gram per Tablespoon. Mix with horseradish and cream to make a horseradish cream sauce for roast beef.

Worcestershire Sauce – Your Keto beef stews and soups will taste wonderful with a splash of Worcestershire sauce. One Tablespoon has 3.3 grams of carbohydrates.

Baking Ingredients

Almond Extract – There are no carbs in almond extract! It gives a nice nutty flavor to Keto Fat Bombs and baking.

Almond Flour – Every type of white or wheat based flour is off limits on the Keto Diet. But you can have almond flour! It's made up of ground almonds and gives a slight nutty taste to baking. For every ¼ cup, you get 6 grams of carbohydrates and 14 grams of the good fats. It is a bit high in carbs, so factor those into your daily Macro percentages.

Baking Powder – Your Keto bread doughs and pizza recipes won't rise without baking powder, so this is an ingredient to have in your kitchen. Baking powder has 1.3 grams of carbohydrates per teaspoon.

Cocoa Powder – High quality unsweetened cocoa powder will make your Keto Fat Bombs and baked goods taste delicious! Just one Tablespoon has 3 grams of carbs.

Coconut Flour – Coconut flour, made from coconuts, is another ingredient to substitute in baking for white flour. That way, you can make Keto breads and doughs. It has 16 grams of carbohydrates and 4 grams of fat per ¼ cup. That's a pretty high carb count, so use it sparingly.

Dark Chocolate – Yes, you can have chocolate on the Ketogenic Diet. Add it to baked goods, Keto hot chocolate, or have a small nibble as a snack when cravings strike. Look for high quality dark chocolate bars that have at least 80% cacao in them and the lowest amount of sugar you can find. Some companies make Keto friendly dark chocolate morsels and chips, too.

Flaxseed Meal – Flax seeds are very low carb and a crunchy topping for Keto salads. Flaxseed meal is an essential baking ingredient for several recipes, so you'll want to have some in your pantry. Two Tablespoons have 4 grams of carbohydrates.

Lemon Extract – Make Keto lemon cookies with carb free lemon extract. That hint of tartness really elevates your baking.

Psyllium Husk Powder – Psyllium husk is a form of fiber made from the husks of the Platago ovata plant's seeds. Psyllium husk powder can be mixed with other flours and baking ingredients to make Keto pizza dough. You probably won't find it in your local grocery store, but it can be in health food stores or purchased online.

Stevia – No white sugar or brown sugar allowed on the Ketogenic Diet. However, you can have a natural substitute. Stevia has 1 gram per 2 teaspoons, so it's okay to add a dash to your morning coffee, afternoon tea, or slip into Keto Fat Bombs. Go easy on the Stevia, but it can help you with sugar cravings.

Vanilla Extract – At less than 1 gram of carbs per teaspoon, you can add delicious vanilla flavor to your Keto Fat Bombs, bullet proof coffee, cookies, and cakes.

Other

Lard – Yep, the old-fashioned pig fat lard. It's full of healthy saturated fats. There are 13 grams of fat per Tablespoon.

MCT oil - This ingredient, called Medium-chain triglyceride oil, might not be found at your grocery store, although some specialty health food stores could carry it. It's easier to digest than other oils, a great source of energy, and supports the hormones in your body.

Olives – Green olives have 2.8 grams of carbohydrates and are packed with amazing good fats, so buy plenty! Black olives are higher in carbs, so stick with green ones only.

Getting Your Pantry Ready for the Keto Lifestyle

Time to give your kitchen a makeover! Ridding your cupboards, fridge, and freezer of carbs, fruits, and sugars is the best beginner tip for starting the Ketogenic Diet. You're able to give yourself a clean slate and start fresh with new foods that actually work with your body.

In this chapter, you've read all about ingredients that are Keto Diet friendly, so those are the only ones to keep. All the rest must go. If you feel guilty about throwing out perfectly good food, then call up a friend or family member and bring it over to them. You can donate canned beans and boxed pastas or grains to your local food bank.

Eating Out on the Keto Diet

Restaurants know that we crave their meals, and they pile on the sugar and carbs. You'd be amazed at how quickly a simple appetizer can derail your best laid plans for weight loss and health. How do you know which restaurants to pick that are Keto Diet friendly?

Take a walk around your neighborhood (or use a smartphone app or local website) to really look at your restaurant options. You'll see fast food places, soup and sandwich shops, pizza joints, international food restaurants, dinner restaurants, and sweets places like bakeries, cafes, and ice cream stands. Look up restaurant menus online to see which options they have that you can use on the Keto Diet.

Here are some general tips to ordering in a restaurant:

- Ask them to remove the bread.
- Crispy means fried and fried means the wrong types of oils and plenty of trans fats. Order grilled instead.
- Portions are way too big. Either share with a friend or ask the restaurant to box up half the meal to take home for lunch the next day.
- Put together several Keto friendly appetizers and sides instead of an entrée. You can choose from soups, salads, grilled meats, spice rubbed fish, and vegetables like broccoli or zucchini.
- "Breaded" is a code word for "coated in bread crumbs." Stay away from carbs.
- Many restaurants have gluten-free options to help you remove carbs. Ask your server.

Basically, when you order in a restaurant, think of the types of Keto friendly meals you make at home. Then, try as closely as possible to replicate those meals.

80% Keto Friendly Restaurants:

Choose these to find great menus filled with plenty of things to eat:

- Breakfast places – Eggs, bacon, sausage, ham, steak, and cheese galore.
- Steak house restaurants – Any protein grilled and served alongside broccoli or cauliflower is a good bet. No baked potatoes.
- Barbecue restaurants – Lots of protein options here: chicken, beef, pork, ham, or even fish. Skip the cornbread and mashed potatoes, and go for the collard greens instead.
- Seafood restaurants – Dip that lobster in butter! You can have any type of fish or shrimp with a Keto veggie side. Make sure it's not breaded.
- Asian restaurants – Thai, Vietnamese, Chinese, Japanese, and other Asian restaurants offer plenty of entrees with no carbs. Hold the rice and noodles.
- French restaurants – All that Brie, butter, heavy cream, shallots, and mushrooms are excellent on a Keto diet.
- Indian restaurants – You won't find any beef dishes, but there are delicious chicken, lamb, and vegetarian options. No rice or naan.

50% Keto Friendly Restaurants:

The following menus have limited Keto options, so you'll have to do a bit of navigating:

- Diners – Skip the dinner rolls and order either steak or chicken dishes with Keto veggie sides.
- Mexican restaurants – Navigate past the corn, beans, rice, and tortillas. Go for the grilled shrimp, salsa, and queso.
- Soup, Salad, and Sandwich places – Try ordering a cup of Keto friendly soup and a side salad. If they have lettuce wraps, go for it.
- Italian restaurants – Difficult, but you can order chicken parmesan with no pasta. Get creative!
- Mediterranean restaurants – Stay away from hidden carbs like pita, barley, quinoa, and couscous.
- Bars and pubs – You'll find lots of potatoes and bread, but you can order chicken wings in a pinch.
- Fast Food Burger Joints – Not easy, but we have faith you can order burgers with no buns!

No – No Restaurants:

Please avoid these on the Keto Diet!

- Pizza restaurants – Everything is served either on top of or alongside bread. Lots of bread.
- Coffee Shops – Turning plain coffee into dessert drinks. Step away from the breakfast pastries!
- Bakeries – Pretty self explanatory. Nothing but sugar and carbs.
- Ice Cream / Dessert places – Sugar, sugar, and more sugar.
- Carnivals – You won't find anything remotely healthy or Keto friendly in fair food. It's all carbs that are battered and fried.
- Movie Theaters – You get three terrible choices: soda, candy, or popcorn. No thanks!

- Sports stadium food – You might be able to get away with ballpark franks without the bun, but that's about it.
- Convenience Stores – Nothing but soda, candy, potato chips, and sugary packaged treats.
- Vending Machines – Just seeing if you're paying attention!

Just because you can't have pizza, baked goods, or pasta, doesn't mean there aren't amazing other options on the Ketogenic Diet! In your first month of eating on this plan, you might want to avoid most of these restaurants, so that you're not tempted to eat something you shouldn't.

Now that you've got your ingredients, your Keto friendly stocked kitchen and have successfully navigated the world of restaurants, how exactly will you be eating each day? In the next chapter, we'll get into the nitty gritty of getting into ketosis: Macros!

Chapter 4:
Come Here And Learn All About It!

Getting started on the Keto Diet is just the first step in an exciting journey! As you saw in the previous chapter, there are foods you can't eat. But you'll feel so good you won't be tempted to order a carb-heavy meal and kick yourself out of ketosis! You'll want to stay in this new metabolic state for life.

There are some basic tenets of the Keto lifestyle that can help you along the way. They're easy to memorize and can be repeated to yourself, similar to mantras.

"No Sugar Today – Feeling Sweet Tomorrow"

You'll get sugar cravings on the Keto diet. But, they do get better with time. If you can say no to a sugary item now, you'll feel sweet and look better tomorrow.

"It's Not About Can't – It's About Don't"

Forget saying, "I can't have carbs." Start saying: "I don't want carbs." It's a subtle, but necessary mindset shift. It'll really help you.

"I'm Just Not Hungry for That"

You can mentally trick your taste buds into finding a particular food distasteful. Some people love licorice; others hate it. Some people hate mushrooms; others love them. Try and mentally trick yourself into just not being hungry for some carb item that'll just sit in your stomach and make you feel sluggish.

You can come up with your own mantras, too. Been suffering from a health problem? Imagine feeling better once Keto has helped reduce your symptoms. Sick and tired of low energy? Create a mantra that focuses on what you want to use your new energy for. When you custom tailor a mantra, you're more likely to remember it.

To remember it even more, take a pen and write out your mantra on a piece of paper. Don't type it. Hand write it. That puts it into your memory.

Know Your Body

Each of us start out wanting to know exactly what state our body is in. When you assess where you are today, right now during the exact moment you're reading this, then that gives you a start point. It's like the first "Start" square on a gameboard. Today is when you'll begin. It also functions as a reference point for the progress you'll make throughout the next few weeks as you transition to this new eating plan.

Think of where you were just one year ago. You've progressed a long way since then. It might not be in the direction you want, but it is a different direction. Diets can be difficult, because they're measured on a longer time frame than many of us want them to be! We want to see results in days, whereas your body operates on a much more elongated calendar. Patience creates results.

So do metrics. Body metrics, specifically. In this beginning state, you're encouraged to get your full physical self assessed. This can be done through a simple physical at your doctor's. Please fill out the following:

Height:

Current Weight:

BMI:

You are also highly HIGHLY encouraged to keep a food diary. Just get a simple notebook from a store and write down everything you eat and drink. Beginning this simple habit is eye-opening.

After you have your numbers and metrics from your doctor visit, what's the next step?

The Keto Mindset

It's not just about numbers, as those of you who've dieted before well know. It also has so much to do with your mindset. While it may come across as mumbo-jumbo, uncovering your personal psychological reasons for why you want to get healthier and more slim and trim, plus your current emotional state, will help you so much later on, when you'll have to face the challenges of this diet (as any diet). Just like a Greek warrior gathering his magic sword and shield from the gods, so, too, will you gather the tools you need to fight against your old impulses, overcome them, and win!

Yes, fighting the carb battle is a battle. So, it is important that we discuss one powerful word:

WHY?

Why do you want to embark on this Ketogenic Diet? Although initially the reason might be that it looks cool, it's a neat fad, cutting out carbs is easier than ever, or whatever, you've got to come up with deeper reasons.

So, why?

Why do you want to succeed on the Keto Diet? Why do you want to start it in the first place? Why do you have strong feelings about this diet, as opposed to another one? Why do you want to be healthier?

It helps to raise your own stakes in this battle. Many people have a near-death experience before they make a radical change – and that's because they've realized there's high stakes involved. If they don't do X, it might harm or even kill them in the long run.

What are your high stakes? If you don't embark on this diet and make it a success, then what's your high stakes reason to keep going? It could be something personal, that you're doing this for you. It could be spiritual, that you feel you were given this physical body from a higher power and you want to treat it better. It could be relational, like you're doing this for your family member, friend, or other loved one. It could be physical, that you're simply sick and tired of being sick and tired. There's only so much you can take!

It would be helpful to write this down in a journal. That is an excellent place to more deeply explore your thoughts. Make it easy on yourself to remember your reason. How about tattooing it on your arm? Just kidding!

But seriously. Discipline comes from strong and compelling reasons. Find a reason stronger than the breadstick sitting on the table in front of you, strong enough to say no to a hundred breadsticks – and you'll find your own diet success.

Keto Diet Tools

You want to transition from a carbohydrate metabolic state to a ketosis metabolic state and stay there. Just because you're low carb doesn't mean your liver is producing ketones. To measure ketosis, there are several tools on the market that you can buy to help you:

- Blood Ketone Monitor
- Breath Ketone Monitor
- Ketone Urine Strips

These three tools can test your blood, breath, or urine. They're easy to test at home by yourself. Your ideal ketone level varies depending on your age, gender, height, weight, and other body factors.

The Blood Ketone Monitor is similar to diabetes insulin testing. Insert the strip into the monitor machine, prick your finger to put blood on the strip, and you'll get a reading pretty quickly. While this is the most expensive method, it's the most accurate method of determining you're in ketosis.

To use a Breath Ketone Monitor, you'll plug the device into a power source, blow on it until the light stops flashing, take a note of the color and how many times it blinks. This takes a bit longer and hasn't been researched as much as the other solutions.

For the Ketone Urine Strips, you'll just pee on a stick, wait about a minute, and then compare the color to the chart on the package. It's the least expensive of the three methods, but don't work after you enter ketosis.

It's up to you which one you prefer using. I recommend the Breath Ketone Monitor, since it isn't painful and it measures those ketones properly.

Ketogenic Diet Macros

I've got good news! No need to count calories on the Ketogenic Diet! You can if you want to. But it's not as important as tracking your Macros. So, we do need to learn how to calculate those.

This diet is made up of three Macronutrients, which are nicknamed Macros:

FATS – PROTEINS – CARBOHYDRATES

Yes, carbs are included. We're not going to eliminate them completely, just reduce them to a tiny percentage.

On a normal balanced diet, which is recommended by USDA nutritional guidelines, you'd be consuming 35% of your daily calories from carbohydrates, 35% of your daily calories from proteins, and about 5% of your daily calories from good fats.

But the Macros on a Ketogenic Diet are much different.

With fats, we're going to increase from 5% all the way up to 70% of your daily calories from good fats. We'll discuss what good fats are below.

With proteins, you'll reduce the 35% down to about 19% protein.

With the carbohydrates, you'll be reducing that 60% down to about 5% - 8% of your daily calories.

So, we're going from this:

5% FATS - 35% PROTEINS – 60% CARBOHYDRATES

To this:

70% FATS – 19% PROTEINS – 5% CARBOHYDRATES

That's your new diet, one that will keep your body in a ketosis state.

How does this break down into counts in grams?

It varies depending on your body factors (gender, age, height, weight, etc.), but in general, you should aim for:

MEN:

208g FATS – 125g PROTEINS – 31g CARBOHYDRATES

WOMEN:

167g FATS – 100g PROTEINS – 25g CARBOHYDRATES

You can find Keto Macro calculators online that give you the exact numbers. My main point is just to have you keep your Macro numbers in mind, especially during your first four weeks of transition. For some, these carb grams might be a bit high for ketosis. That's why you should be using the Ketone monitors mentioned above to make absolutely sure.

Now, let's talk about each Macro and what it's for in your body!

Let's Start with Protein

Protein is one of your body's most essential nutrients. It's also delicious, too – roasted, baked, and grilled meats get your mouth watering for a reason. There are two types of protein: animal and plant. On the Ketogenic Diet, your plant intake is reduced because many vegetables and fruits have too many carbs. So, you're primarily going to get your protein from animal sources: meat, fish, seafood, eggs, and high protein dairy foods.

What does protein do in your body? It is a general repairman and handyman. It repairs and builds tissue, makes enzymes, makes hormones, and builds bones, muscle, cartilage, skin, and blood. It also gives you energy. Your brain needs a lot of protein for basic mental functions, too.

While protein is essential, it's not the amazing nutrient that's frequently advertised by food manufacturers. Most Americans consume too much protein, trying to get to that nationally recommended 35% amount. To get into and stay in ketosis, protein is important, but not as important as fat. Excess protein can also be stored as excess weight in your cells, so too much of a good thing is, well, not a good thing.

On the Ketogenic Diet, we'll reduce your protein amount to between 19% and 22% of your diet. It's easy to go overboard with the protein. Meats do have high percentages of good fats, though.

Keep your protein calorie counts a bit lower than you're used to. The Keto Diet is not a high protein diet.

The Truth Behind Carbohydrates

Carbohydrates are made up of the same three atoms as fatty acids: carbon, hydrogen, and oxygen. By themselves, these don't seem like bad chemical components, and they're not. When we think carbs, we think bread or pasta or cereal, right? That's because you see the high carbohydrate count on these foods.

Carbohydrates are a group of sugars, starches, and cellulose called saccharides. Starch and sugar are basically the two most important carbohydrates in nutrition.

There are four chemical groups of saccharides: the monosaccharides, disaccharides, oligosaccharides, and polysaccharides. Those are pretty big chemical names, but we're primarily going to focus on how they function in your body.

Sugars and Starches

Polysaccharides store energy in your cells, in the form of starch and glycogen. It's the starch present in foods like potatoes, rice, and wheat that eventually becomes too much stored energy in your body, resulting in weight gain. Sugars have the "ose" suffix, and you'll see them as sucrose (table sugar), fructose (fruit sugar), and glucose (blood sugar). Some people are lactose intolerant, so they can't have milk sugar. There's also cellulose, which is plant sugar, and we'll talk more about that below.

Glycogen is the other type of energy stored in your cells, and it's also a carbohydrate. It's primarily found in both your liver and your muscles.

Carbs Are Actually Sugars

So, when you're walking by the bakery section in the grocery store or the goodies in the snack aisle, just remember that all of those carbohydrates are actually sugars that will add weight. They don't burn off the weight you're trying to lose, either.

It's so tempting, because we live in such a carb loving and carb heavy culture. You bypass them in the grocery store all the time. You drive by fast food restaurants advertising sandwiches and fries, you can barely order an entrée without carbs, every convenience store sells potato chips, and entire cuisines like Italian and Mexican are built on carbohydrate foundations of pasta, bread dough, and rice.

But they all just become glucose sugar molecules in your body and contribute to weight gain.

Leave the carbohydrates on the shelf!

Fat Doesn't Necessarily Make You Fat

Now, let's talk about your number one Macro: fat.

Fat can mean so many different things. It's not just about making you fat. It's also about what fatty acids inside the fats are good for you. And many of them are! These are the fats your liver needs to break down and make ketones.

Yes, it's weird to think eating a high fat diet helps you burn fat. But it's absolutely true.

At the chemical level, a fat is composed of two different kinds of smaller molecules. One of them is glycerol, and the other is fatty acids. Glycerol is a simple compound that's colorless, odorless, has a sweet taste and is non-toxic to humans. The fatty acids are long acids made up of chains of atoms that include different combinations of carbon, oxygen, and hydrogen atoms.

Did you know that fatty acids aren't actually found in humans naturally? We get them from our diet, and they're one of the primary sources of fuel for most of our cells.

The good fats also break down more slowly than carbohydrates in your digestive tract. That means you'll feel full longer.

Good Fats and Bad Fats

The food industry is confusing enough without having to explain the difference between good fats and bad fats. While you're on the Ketogenic Diet, you want to stick to the 'good' fats, which we'll talk about in this chapter. We'll also discuss the 'bad' fats and why they're bad.

As a general guideline, you'll want to stick to eating fats that are naturally occurring in plants, animals, and seafoods. Processed fats are created in food product factories to add taste and flavor to many foods, including margarine, fried foods, and processed cheese. Eating all natural fats is basically the way to go.

It's important to know the difference between good and bad fats, because the good ones will have a positive effect on your body and keep you in ketosis. The bad fats will have a negative effect on your body and contribute towards not just weight gain, but circulatory problems like blocked arteries and even heart disease. Bad fats aren't processed by the body and used as fuel the same way the good fats are.

So, let's discuss the differences and examine them at a chemical level.

Good Fats

The two good fats are saturated fats and monounsaturated fats. Natural polyunsaturated fats can also be added to this category. They are better for your body because of the amount of chains of fatty acids found in them. What are they and how do they help your body?

Saturated Fat

This type of fat is one that contains a high proportion of fatty acid molecules without double bonds. These double bonds link individual carbon atoms to hydrogen atoms, which changes the chemical properties. The reason they're called saturated is because the molecules are saturated with hydrogen atoms. They are solid at room temperature and have higher melting points. The fats from animals are mostly saturated, which is why you'll find saturated fats in animal products like meats and dairy. Saturated fats get a bad rap because they can also be found in processed foods. We'll advise you on which saturated fats to consume in the next chapter.

Monounsaturated Fat

The second type of good fat for the Keto Diet is monounsaturated fat. It also contains a high proportion of fatty acid molecules, but these come with just one double bond (where the prefix 'mono' comes in) that link carbon atoms to hydrogen ones. At room temperature, they are liquids and either semi-solid or solid when refrigerated.

When your cells start to use monounsaturated fats for fuel, there's not as many calories as the saturated fats. These are good fats because they protect against cardiovascular disease and are better fuel for your cells.

Bad Fats

The fats to avoid are the processed polyunsaturated fats and the trans fats. You've probably heard of these two bad guys. They have become not just diet enemies, but health enemies as well.

Processed Polyunsaturated Fats

Polyunsaturated fats are similar to the monounsaturated fats above, in that they contain a high proportion of fatty acid molecules. But these ones have more than one double bond between carbon and hydrogen atoms. While carbon and hydrogen don't sound like a bad pairing, in this case, too much of a good thing becomes a bad thing. We listed the processed version of these fats as the real culprit, but naturally occurring polyunsaturated fats are okay to eat. The processed version is often found in certain oils, like corn oil, soybean oil, and other fatty foods like margarine. Naturally occurring polyunsaturated fats are encouraged for you to eat. You might know them better as Omega-3 and Omega-6 fatty acids.

Trans Fats

Trans fat is the nickname for trans-fatty acids, which are the worst kind of fats. They're so bad they're banned in restaurants around the world. They've been around since the 1950s, with the rise of quick frying and the food product industry. Trans fats come from better unsaturated fats, but they have even more double bonds. They directly contribute towards raising your LDL lipoprotein levels, which is called bad cholesterol, lowering your good cholesterol, and directly contributing towards diseases. Trans fats are used to make foods taste better and have a longer shelf life. Plenty of bad foods on any diet are full of trans fats, including microwaved butter popcorn, carnival fried foods, and frozen breakfast sandwiches.

As long as you stay away from these bad fats, you should do just fine!

What About Vegetables?

It's a myth that eating certain vegetables help you lose weight. Their carbohydrate contents are simply too high. To eat some of these vegetables would be the equivalent of having a slice of toast, which is also forbidden.

Yes, it's bizarre that high carbohydrate foods like potatoes and carrots are unhealthier for you than full fat butter! But when it comes down to the cellular differences in how your body actually processes carbohydrates vs. the good fats, it becomes obvious.

Cellulose is present in the cell walls of all plant materials, and it is also known as fiber to help maintain your healthy digestive system. But cellulose is also a carbohydrate, just like starch and sugar. Some vegetables, like potatoes and corn, have too much starch in relation to their cellulose levels. That's why they're not considered as part of the Ketogenic Diet. Those carbohydrate molecules will be too much stored energy in your body and will also kick you out of ketosis.

Forget Conventional Nutritional Information

In order to have success on the Ketogenic Diet, you're going to have to forget a lot of the conventional nutritional information that you've learned over the years. The Food Pyramid has too many carbohydrates and doesn't work, the USDA Food Nutrition Guidelines don't take into account how your body actually processes nutrients, and fats aren't your number one diet enemy. Whole grains aren't as healthy for you as you think. A grain is still a grain, and grains are made up of carbohydrates.

The Ketogenic Diet has its own rules for how your body really works when in a ketosis metabolic state.

The reason we went into so much detail about how your body processes fats, carbohydrates, starches, and sugars is because ...

That's essentially what's going on at a cellular level when you eat foods on the Ketogenic Diet.

Stick to these three Macros and their percentages:

70% FATS – 19% PROTEINS – 5% CARBOHYDRATES

These Macros switch your body from that carbohydrate metabolic state to the ketosis metabolic state.

Right now, whenever you eat something, your body is using the same old energy storing techniques. Think of your body as a warehouse. Shipments of new carbohydrates, fats, proteins, and other molecules are continually coming into the warehouse. Whenever new carbohydrates come in, a few of those sugars and starches are used for energy. That's the brief burst of craziness you get after eating a candy bar or the temporary 'sugar high.' But mostly, the rest of those carbohydrates are stored in the warehouse, not to be used again. You eat something else with carbohydrates in it, and the cycle repeats itself. A fraction is used for energy, and the rest is stored in your cells.

Too much stored energy results in the weight gain you're experiencing. For those of you who've tried exercising to take off the weight, you become frustrated because spending 30 minutes at the gym four times a week isn't going to stop the storage warehouse cycle. It isn't going to magically switch your body from storing energy to burning energy.

But, being in ketosis does do that!

The Keto Diet basically switches your body from an energy storage container to an energy burning machine.

That's what we're going for in this book.

Creating Ketones For Weight Loss

Once you've entered a state of ketosis and your liver is producing ketones, you'll notice the weight will start to come off. It's almost effortless, and doesn't require any additional exercise (although some is recommended).

The best thing you can do for your body and especially your liver, is to monitor your Macros on the Ketogenic Diet. Stick to your high fat percentage, moderate protein percentage, and very low carbohydrate percentage.

Chapter 5:
Your First 4 Weeks on The Keto Diet

When getting started on the Keto Diet, this chapter will be your nitty gritty guide to making it work! We're going to go through everything you should be eating, doing, and monitoring, making this transition as easy and enjoyable as possible.

I know you feel you've got plenty of information already, you've got the foods you can eat, there's a meal plan in two chapters, and you can just fly off on your own, right? You'll be just fine.

Hold up there! Please be patient with yourself and your body and follow these steps. Remember your body is changing its entire metabolic state. That's a big transition. Take it slow for the first four weeks, and you'll be assured of greater success in the long run.

Week One

Yay, you're starting the diet! Lots of support and encouragement from me here. You're armed with quite a few tools, including your list of foods you can eat, the foods you cannot have, the meal plans, the recipes, and at least one monitoring device for ketosis. You feel ready to set off on this new diet adventure. The beginning is filled with both drive and enthusiasm.

However, you could also be experiencing a bit of the trepidatious fear of the unknown. What's life without bread, pasta, rice, potatoes, and corn? Is this diet really all it's cracked up to be? Will my body respond just like all those others who've been on the Ketogenic Diet? What will be my results?

Yep, lots of questions. That's why it's helpful to keep a food journal or diary to track this transition period.

Dealing with Hunger

Up until now, when you've been in the mood for a snack, you've reached for something with carbs in it. Potato chips, pretzels, popcorn, maybe a piece of toast, or some crackers.

But when those items are off the menu, what do you substitute them with? Hopefully, you followed the 'cleaning the pantry' suggestions in the Foods to Eat chapter above. You do have plenty of snack options – cheese, nuts, hard boiled eggs, fresh veggies with tahini.

Hungry for something sweet? Try a cup of tea with a pinch of Stevia in it, or by making one of the Fat Bombs in the recipes chapter. Having a sweet tooth on the Ketogenic Diet does get better as the days go by. Make sure you're getting enough fat, and that will help.

Carb and Sugar Withdrawal

As part of dealing with hunger pangs, you might go through carbohydrate withdrawals. This is definitely natural and expected. Eating all of those sugars affected your brain in such a profound chemical way that it's like you've been on a stimulating drug! The symptoms of withdrawal include:

- Rampant sugar cravings

- Obsessing over sweet or carb foods
- Mood swings
- Dizziness
- Irritability
- Fatigue

Luckily, you'll only feel these symptoms for a few days. By the end of the first week, those cravings and these negative feelings will be much subsided. Then you'll emerge from it being better than ever, your blood sugar will stabilize and calm down, and your overall well being will be much improved. I went through it, too.

Pass the Salt

Keep that salt shaker handy during your first week on the Keto Diet. You were probably getting a great deal of your daily recommended allowance of sodium from carb foods, like potato chips and French fries.

By limiting your carbohydrates to around 30 grams per day, you're not eating large amounts of glucose. That means your body's not producing as much insulin. However, insulin not only is in conjunction with your blood sugar, but also your blood sodium levels by helping sodium get absorbed into the body. Without it, you'd just pee out the salt. It is a mineral, after all!

Having low insulin while in ketosis means that you're going to be urinating out much more sodium. This means you're also losing lots of electrolytes. So, you need to increase your salt intake. Aim for between 2000 mg and 4000 mg per day.

Fortunately, there's many yummy solutions: salty cheeses, salty nuts, salted meats, salted fish, salted butter, and sprinkling salt on salads. You can sip on salty chicken or beef broth between meals, too. This will also help to relieve lots of those carb withdrawal symptoms discussed above.

Keep your salt intake nice and high during not just your first week, but the entire time you're in ketosis on the Keto Diet. Don't forget to stay hydrated, too!

Week One Foods:

In addition to your salty foods, you'll want to slowly ease into the diet within your first week by choosing different foods and meals that are no carb.

MCT Oil

One of the foods discussed above was MCT Oil. It's worth it to pick up a bottle of this unusual supplement. MCT (medium-chain triglycerides) oil is found in coconut oil or it can be purchased separately at a health food store or online. MCT oil is a fat similar to olive oil that can be rapidly absorbed. It goes right to your liver, which is either immediately used for energy or converted right into ketones. Start with a lower dosage to see how it interacts with your body, and then gradually increase.

It supplies plenty of good nutrients your body needs for the transition. Right when you're fresh out of bed is when it can work the best. Keep up this practice for at least 14 days straight, and you'll achieve ketosis even faster.

More Butter … and Then More

One of the many changes is wrapping your mind around the previous off limits foods you're now encouraged to eat. When cooking, reach for the butter. Put lots of butter (and salt!) on vegetables. Dip shellfish like crab, shrimp, or lobster into butter. Create a garlic butter sauce for fish or chicken. Butter is amazing and will help you get through the first week on the Keto Diet.

Drink Bullet Proof Coffee

What's bullet proof coffee? It's a simple cup of Joe that's been jolted with extra Keto friendly ingredients to turn it into a caffeinated and high performance drink. One serving has a whopping 28.5 fat grams, and only 1 gram of carbohydrates. You'll need 1 cup of black coffee, 1 Tablespoon of high quality grass fed unsalted butter, 1 Tablespoon coconut or MCT oil, ½ Tablespoon heavy cream, and ½ teaspoon vanilla extract. Mix everything in a blender or by hand and drink. It gives you so many good fats and is an excellent healthy start to your day. Pairing it with a high fat, low carb breakfast is one of the best ways to start on your Keto Diet. I also include a second recipe for Almond Bullet Proof Coffee in this book I think you'll love, too!

Nuts About Nuts

I've mentioned eating nuts several times to help you get through your first week. They provide a salty, meaty crunch as a snack food, plus they're packed with good fats and very low or no carbohydrates. Macadamia nuts, almonds, and walnuts can be mixed with low carb chocolate chips and seeds to create a yummy snack mix that will see you through your first week.

Cheesy and Delicious

Cheese really is delicious. You can snack on cheddar, goat cheese, cottage cheese, Colby Jack, mozzarella sticks, or any other creamy cheeses in the Foods to Eat chapter above. Having a few pieces of cheese boosts your fat intake. Don't forget melted cheese, too. Sprinkle shredded cheese on top of salads, chicken, or ground beef dishes. You can also create baked cheese dips for veggies.

Week One Tips

Hopefully, these tips and tricks will help you get through your first week on the Keto Diet. You might see a pound or two of initial weight loss, but you might not. This first week is more about slowly but steadily changing your mindsets around foods, increasing your fat intake, and trying new ways to get your ideal Macros through MCT oil and bullet proof coffee.

As another practical tip, read through the recipes in this book and make sure you've purchased the items you need to make all the meals. You'll need mini muffin tins or candy molds for the Fat Bombs, a blender for smoothies, and it helps to have a large crock pot for busy week nights. That way, by next week, you'll be able to make all the recipes.

It's not a race, so go slow. Your main objective is to reduce those carbohydrates and rid your home of them, and steadily increase your fat intake. Stock your cupboards with new foods and start experimenting with the recipes. It's helpful to start on a weekend day, so you have more time to go Keto for a full day.

Week Two

Good! You got through Week One! You knew that was going to be the hardest, and for some of you, the cravings and withdrawal symptoms were not easy to get through. But, you've made it – and this week is when your diet can start to change your body in new ways and better than you thought possible.

How does it do that?

Well, you're going to start seeing results. Physical results that come from changing to such a low carb lifestyle. The initial pounds that you lose this second week will first come from water weight loss. That is because glycogen from those carbohydrates you were previously eating was stored with H2O water cells throughout your body. You'll notice a drop in weight and a general feeling of lightness after the water weight is shed. Don't expect it to be too much, but it could be noticeable.

However, if this water weight loss doesn't happen, that's also normal. Not to worry! You might not have had that issue in your body. Each person will have a different range of experiences within the first two weeks of going Ketogenic.

Micromanage Your Macros

What truly is the most important thing you should do this second week is to watch your Macros very closely. By now, you should have calculated the exact grams using an online Macros calculator or by going off the guidelines in the previous chapter. This is when you've got to apply some of that discipline to track what you're eating and keep the Macros in your mind at all times.

Fortunately, I've made this super easy on you! Just follow the four-week meal plans in this book! You get two of them, either a regular meal plan or one for busy 30 minute meals. Week Two is an excellent time to start following that meal plan to the letter. The recipes for the meals are also in this book, as well as grocery lists. Please use these tools to your full advantage.

You'll also want to keep monitoring your ketone production using the blood, breath, or urine. Make sure you're not eating that many carbs. Those grams add up quickly.

It's also normal to not feel all that hungry as your body shifts. Just make sure you're getting enough calories and try not to skip meals or try drastic low calorie rations. It's okay to eat this much fat!

The good news is, once you stick to the Macros ratios and keep your grams consistent, it will happen eventually. Your body has this ability to go into ketosis, so keep at it.

The Keto 'Flu'

Since the Ketogenic Diet has become more popular, many dieters on it have talked about what's affectionately nicknamed the Keto Flu. It's not the real flu or influenza, in that there's no virus or bug you caught.

The Keto Flu is a collection of flu-like symptoms many experience after they start this new eating plan. This flu only lasts a few days and shouldn't be enough to call out sick from work or have to miss important appointments. It's simply your body's way of letting you know it's changing metabolic cycles.

When you have the Keto Flu, the first symptom you'll notice will be tiredness. That comes from the switch in metabolism. You also might get a headache and have other mental ailments like difficulty concentrating and brain fog. That's because your brain has been using glycogen for fuel and is now switching to ketones. Your brain requires a massive amount of protein and calories, so it's in essence pulling resources and trying to search for alternative fuel sources. The change in calorie source can also make you irritable, for the same reason being hungry can. You'll also have to urinate more, since your insulin levels are dropping.

While the Keto Flu isn't pleasant while you're experiencing it, count that as a good sign. Your body is effectively switching gears. Within a few days, your body will get the idea that there aren't more glucose or other sugar sources of fuel coming in, and it's time to switch to using the fat stores.

Most people do just fine with this Week Two transition. But, if you're having difficulty with the Keto Flu, read below.

Keto Flu Remedies

Replenishing Electrolytes and Salt

You're losing electrolytes because your insulin levels are dropping. So, slice up some lemons in water and drink that to rehydrate yourself and get those electrolyte levels up again. If the Keto Flu persists, that's a good indication that you're not hydrated enough. Get as much water as you can.

You'll also want to increase your salt intake. Warm up regular sodium (not low sodium) chicken broth or consommé and sip that throughout the day.

Replenishing both your electrolytes and salt will also help with another Keto Flu problem: muscle cramps. Your muscles are also attempting to switch from glycogen as fuel to fat as fuel, and that can cause them to shrink and contract. Muscle cramps might keep you awake at night. Drink as much water as you can and especially water with lemon to make sure you're getting the nutrients you need.

Due to this, you'll find you have to urinate much more frequently! Stay near a bathroom and try not to schedule any long trips or other situations where you can't have access to a restroom.

Bad Breath

Low carbohydrate diets can cause bad breath. It isn't an oral hygiene issue; your digestive system and liver are to blame. It's the ketones your liver emits that are causing the breath, which is why you can measure ketosis through the breath.

To combat this, brush and floss more frequently. Mint is an excellent remedy for bad breath, and chocolate works for some people as well. You can purchase a mint gel or use actual freshly washed mint leaves to rub around the gums and help freshen your breath. Mouth wash can also help. The breath problems do subside after you're fully in ketosis.

The Keto Rash

If your Keto Flu also comes with an overwhelming new sense of itchiness, then you also have the Keto Rash, too. It's a condition that's not dangerous and is called *prurigo pigmentosa*. You may experience some small itchy, raised skin lesions that vary in color between reddish pink to light brown. Yes, they itch. They're not life-threatening, dangerous, or should cause alarm. I just want you to be aware of them. It can increase in intensity from a few spots to a large rash spread over the skin. It does go away after a couple of weeks, and you can use talc-free baby powder to help stop the itch. The ketones are the main cause, so give your body time to adjust to this new diet.

<u>Feast on Good Fats</u>

Increase your fat consumption as well. Make yourself several batches of the Fat Bombs recipes in this book and make sure you're eating plenty of those. Snack on full fat cheeses, nuts, and hard boiled eggs. Track your fat gram Macros.

<u>No Going to the Gym</u>

In addition to eating better and staying hydrated, slow down on your physical activity. It puts a strain on your body to make this transition and exercise at the same time. This is only temporary and just until the Keto Flu symptoms pass away. Then you can return to your favorite high energy workout schedule.

<u>Catch More Zzzzs</u>

Just like when you went through puberty, your body is going through major changes in this early transition period towards ketosis. As a result, you may feel very tired. Some minor insomnia and night time sleeplessness is to be expected. Schedule in an extra nap or two into your day, if you can. Get in plenty of sleep, and that will not only help the Keto Flu symptoms go away, but you'll also feel more refreshed, too.

To help with sleeplessness, try taking a natural sleep aid supplement that has ingredients like Melatonin, valerian root, or chamomile. Eat some turkey just before bed time, which has the tryptophan in it to help lull you to sleep. You can also drink an herbal tea.

Week Two Tips

By week two, you should be fully on your Macros, watching those like a hawk, and keeping track of your grams and percentages. You might feel the Keto Flu symptoms, but stay on the diet.

If you've been sneaking a bit of carbs here and there during this Week Two and are in 'ketosis limbo,' where you're not exactly feeling well but you're not in full ketosis, then there's a good chance your Keto Flu symptoms will stick around longer. Unfortunately, there's no other remedy than to kick those carbs to the curb! This is not a 'cheat day' diet like some others. You really do have to slash your carb count.

Week Three

Congratulations for getting through the first two weeks of the Keto Diet! Those beginning 14 days were going to be some of the toughest, so getting over that is a reason to celebrate. If you did experience the Keto Flu, those symptoms should be starting to subside. If they're not, just read over the list of remedies above and drink as much water with lemon as you can.

This is also a good time to invest in a Keto Breath Monitor or Keto Blood Monitor, if you haven't already done so. The Ketosis Urine Strips only help during the transition. Once you're in ketosis, check your breath or blood every two or three days.

By Week Three, you should also be very familiar with how to count and calculate your Macros in each meal. If you've not started to follow the meal plans in the book, then please do so. Don't make this diet too hard on yourself! Just grocery shop for the ingredients, cook the dishes, and enjoy the new balance of flavors present in each meal.

Weight Loss

For most newbie Keto Dieters, it's really Week Three where they start to see the weight loss. You might even see several pounds come off within these first three weeks. Once your body has gotten the message that it should be in ketosis, that's when the magic happens.

Have fun tracking your weight loss! Set up a calendar with goal weights and rewards. When you've hit five pounds lost, treat yourself to something small. When you reach ten pounds lost, reward yourself again. Keep up the positive reinforcement, so you have something to look forward to. Don't forget to take "before" and "after" pictures, too. Show off your progress. You deserve it!

Boosting Fat Intake

You've become very familiar with the foods you can and cannot eat! You've probably also gone out to restaurants by now and (hopefully) bypassed all that bread and pasta to go for the Keto approved meals.

Now, it's time to make sure that you're keeping your fat intake nice and high. If the day is passing by and you haven't eaten enough fat grams, then reach for another Fat Bomb, piece of cheese, extra slice of bacon, or a dosage of the MCT oil. It really is that important.

Week Three Tips

With the Keto Flu symptoms under control and ketosis finally achieved by watching your Macros and tracking using a monitor, you're well on your way towards being successful as a Keto Dieter.

The best tip this week is just to follow a meal plan to the letter. You can use the ones in this book, or you can make up your own if you feel confident enough! But make sure it's one that inspires you to stick with it. It's one thing to have a low carb meal plan; it's another to eat those meals each day.

Another excellent Week Three tip is to track your weight loss. That will help inspire you as well!

Week Four

If you weren't out of the Keto Flu last week, this is when those icky symptoms finally disappear. Your body has now successfully transitioned from a carbohydrate metabolic state to a ketosis metabolic state! You've got your Keto Monitor and are making sure you're staying in ketosis. You've also been cooking and eating Keto meals, ordering Keto items in restaurants, and even experienced some initial weight loss, too.

Now, you're going to start seeing all those benefits we've been talking about in this book! Your hard work will start to pay off, and you'll experience:

- Better Mental Clarity
- More Energy – some even call it 'lung bursting' energy!
- More Weight Loss
- Increased Sense of Well Being
- Stabilized Moods

- Stabilized Blood Sugar

The Ketogenic Diet has worked for thousands of people who've struggled through the first three weeks, only to get to Week Four and say, "Okay, now I get it! This is what everyone's been talking about!"

Intermittent Fasting

Once you've gotten the hang of the entire Keto diet lifestyle, you can try intermittent fasting. Intermittent fasting is a great way to jolt your body into ketosis. The meal plans in Chapter 7 provide you with plenty of daily food options. But, you're also encouraged to fast one day a week if you're able to, or skip a meal here and there. While fasting, remember to consume plenty of water and help yourself to a cup of bone broth if you're feeling hungry.

Keto in the Kitchen

While Week Four is full of rewards, it also has one potential pitfall: this diet can get repetitive for people who don't cook or aren't as comfortable cooking. That's perfectly understandable! Cooking can seem like just one more chore to add to your busy life.

But, with YouTube videos, television cooking shows, and a little time to devote to your new hobby, you'll grow to like cooking. Here are tips to have fun being Keto in your own kitchen:

- Watch YouTube videos on how to prepare vegetables, and just start practicing. Learn to slice and dice onions, tomatoes, and other veggies.
- With baking, you have to follow recipes and measure everything exactly.
- But with cooking, you can add a little more seasoning or substitute for an ingredient. There's a lot more leeway.
- Become familiar with your oven's temperature. Some ovens are colder than others, so a dish will take longer to cook.
- Clean as you go! While waiting for a pan to heat up, wipe down the counter. Cooking is much more enjoyable in a clean kitchen.
- Learn what flavors go together. Each cuisine (Italian, Mexican, French, Indian, Thai, etc.) has their own core ingredients.

With a little practice and following the recipes, you'll be making Keto recipes in no time. It gets easier and quicker!

I really like to cook! It makes my house smell good, I like the different sounds of meat sizzling or cheese bubbling, and it's quite a sensory experience. Plus, at the end, you get a delicious meal that makes you lose weight, live healthier, and feel better. What's not to love?

Week Four Tips

Week Four is all about getting past the Keto Flu and turning the corner towards a better future on the Keto Diet. You'll stop feeling deprived of carbs and start feeling great because you're seeing the results.

The best tip this week is to make the recipes, stick to the meal plans, and try new dishes. Treat the Keto Diet as an exploration of new flavors and ingredients that you might not have tried before. The average American diet is pretty bland. The ho-hum ingredients are boosted with sugar and carbs to make them taste better.

But when you choose better ingredients and then put them in improved recipes? That's when you'll start to fall in love with your new eating plan.

So, sit down, buckle in, and enjoy the Keto ride!

Something extra

If it please thee

Ok enough with the attempt at high English literature

The reason for this break over here is simply because I wanted to check in with you what you have learnt so far in all these chapters.

If you have taken away 1 single useful thing of value or learnt something that you thought was nice and helpful, could you please help a friend out and leave a review over in amazon?

It's totally great that you are sharing with folks about the book and this will then help more folks to know about what you know too!

Thank you so much!

Chapter 6:
Proven Tips for Staying in Ketosis

In addition to following your first four weeks on the Ketogenic Diet in the previous chapter, this chapter is all about helping you on this diet. We're going to troubleshoot some frequently stated issues that dieters have had and offer solutions that have worked. So, no matter if you're just starting out and struggling or have been in Keto for six months and need a boost, let's get you back on track and make this a success!

Common Issues with the Ketogenic Diet

Not Getting Into Ketosis

Being stuck in 'ketosis limbo' is no fun, even when you're trying to eat as low carb as possible and following the meal plans in the next chapter. Make sure you're out of ketosis by checking with a Keto Monitor your blood, breath, or urine.

With this issue, it all comes down to numbers. Specifically, your Macros numbers. Track each of your Macros (fats – proteins – carbohydrates) and calculate your grams and percentages every day. Watch your food intake for these three, and write down absolutely everything you eat, including all beverages and serving portions, too.

With this, you'll also watch out for gluconeogenesis, a fancy term for your liver making new sugars and using amino acids for energy rather than ketones. This happens when you're eating too much protein. That's why it's important to track this Macro. Try reducing your protein intake by a couple of grams and measure your ketones again with a Keto Monitor.

Food manufacturers stuff hidden carbs and sugars into so many items. You'll have to keep a diligent eye on food labels and make sure you're not consuming anything you're not supposed to. Even a few extra grams makes a big difference. Try to stay within 30 grams of net carbs a day (give or take a gram or two).

Keep a detailed food diary, calculate your Macros, tweak and refine your diet as needed, and you'll get back into ketosis.

The Difference Between Net Carbs and Full Carbs

Curious about the difference between net carb count and gross carb count?

In order to easily calculate the net carbs in a recipe, subtract the insoluble fiber from the total carbohydrate and total fiber counts. We do this because fiber is technically not a carbohydrate. It's the portion of plant derived food that isn't completely broken down by the digestive enzymes in your stomach and intestines. Insoluble fiber doesn't dissolve in water. It's made of non-starch polysaccharides, which means it's not a starch or a carb.

Next, take a look at the sugar alcohol content. If the total sugar alcohol content exceeds 5 grams, subtract half of that number from the total carb count. That yields your net carbs.

Online nutritional calculators are free, easy to use resources that will help keep your carb count low. If you're not losing weight or staying in ketosis, try calculating your full gross carbs. You might be eating too many. Let your body adapt, and then you can slowly switch back to calculating your net carbs.

Insufficient Fat Intake

We talked previously in this book about how 'fat' doesn't make you fat. But this mindset is so deep in American culture, that it can be difficult to keep buying and eating products with good fats in them. You subconsciously avoid them because you don't want to get fat!

But on the Keto Diet, fat is your number one Macro, and you must consume a lot of it. If you have a concern that fats aren't healthy, refer back to Chapter 4 and re-read the section on good fats / bad fats. To ensure that you're eating the healthiest good fats, stick with the monounsaturated fats instead. This does mean you're cutting out the foods that have incredible flavor and taste, since it's the saturated fat that's the yummiest!

I encourage you to follow the meal plans in the next chapter, because each day gives you plenty of fat grams and satisfies the Keto Diet intake. Keep a food diary and track this Macro, since it's the most important one!

Eating Too Much or Too Often

Just because I heartily encourage you to eat lots of fat grams and a good amount of protein doesn't mean you should go crazy and consume lots of food at once!

I'm of the belief that restaurants have contributed to most Americans not really understanding proper portion and serving sizes. For example, a serving of chicken is 3-4 ounces, the size of a deck of cards. But order a chicken entrée in a restaurant, and they serve at least double that. Oh, and forget about burger sizes! Those are enormous. Portions are just way too big. Watch your serving sizes on the Keto Diet. Eating too much of any one thing, but especially carbs or protein, will keep you out of ketosis.

When you first start on the Keto Diet, you'll be eating the regular 3 meals a day, plus a drink, snack, or dessert. But being in ketosis helps reduce a ravenous appetite, so don't be surprised if you drop back down to just 2 or 2 ½ meals a day. It naturally suppresses your hunger.

Your Body's Carbohydrate Tolerance

The reason the Macros percentages are approximate, is because everybody has a slightly different carbohydrate tolerance. You might be doing the Keto Diet with a friend and notice he or she is able to eat 10 more grams of carbs than you and still lose weight. Consuming lots of carbohydrates also has resulted in metabolic damage to the body, but that exists in varying degrees. Your friend could have less damage and a better tolerance than you, or vice versa.

The good news is, the longer you're keeping your body in a ketosis state, the more it adapts to such a low carb diet. You might even find you can sneak in an extra gram or two of carbohydrates and still stay in ketosis. However, don't cheat for at least your first two months. Give your body time to fully adapt.

Why Aren't I Losing Weight?

Yes, it can be frustrating to pass up on all those carby, sugary treats you used to eat all the time, and the numbers on the scale aren't budging! It's a slippery slope towards feeling deprived, which then can cause you to throw up your hands and make a beeline for the nearest piece of bread. Stop!

Consider this for a moment. Your body could actually be in perfect balance. The energy you're consuming is on one side of the scale and the energy you're expending is on the other side. If those two numbers equal each other, that means no weight loss. You will gain the health benefits in this equalized state. To increase weight loss, try a little bit of exercise (but only after your Keto Flu symptoms have gone away). A few daily walks around the block could be all it takes to tip the scale in your favor.

You may not be fully in ketosis, either. Check with one of the Keto Monitors to be sure. If you're still experiencing the Keto Flu, that's the culprit. Return to diligently tracking your Macros.

Help! My Cholesterol is Out of Whack!

So, you've been to the doctor, they've done their tests, and now they've told you that both your HDL and LDL cholesterol levels have risen considerably. No cause for alarm! About one third of Keto Dieters experience this.

However, cholesterol is actually used by the body as a substance for repair and healing, similar to protein. It's a general handyman. So, when your LDL cholesterol levels rise, that could be a response to more repair going on in your body. That's a good thing! Your body is now working to repair the metabolic damage from eating too many carbohydrates.

So, not to worry about cholesterol levels. It doesn't mean plaque is building up in your arteries or your organs are at risk. It just indicates your LDL cholesterol 'handy men' are hard at work fixing you.

The Keto Lifestyle

If you fall out of ketosis, it isn't the end of the world. You can return to tracking your Macros, saying no to carbs and sugars, and reaching for more healthy fats at any time.

You've now been fully prepped and informed about what it takes to make the Keto Diet a success. It's more of a lifestyle, in that you'll be spending each day preparing and eating a whole new way. The Keto Diet favors those who stick with it over a long period of time. Your body will become more and more adapted, you'll lose weight, you'll feel better, and you'll be healthier, too.

Now, it's time to give you one of the most helpful tools in this book: a meal plan. In the next chapter, you'll get 8 weeks of meals, split into two different meal plans. That's 56 days of Keto Diet eating!

I want nothing but success for you on this health journey.

Chapter 7:
The 4 Week Meal Plans

Having these two excellent meal plans in this chapter ensures your success on the Ketogenic Diet. You get two plans, each for four weeks:

1. Basic Meal Plan – Four weeks of breakfast, lunch, snack, dinner, and dessert options.
2. 30-Minute Meal Plan – Four weeks of quick meals for busy families and households. Food on the table in 30 minutes or less!

You'll see some recipe overlap between the two meal plans. Both are entirely Ketogenic Diet friendly. Please see the Appendix for the grocery lists for both meal plans, split into two-week intervals to make it easier and cheaper for shopping.

The Basic Meal Plan will help you as you begin your journey into the Keto lifestyle! Each day includes three meals plus one snack, dessert, or drink. Each recipe lists the calories and Macros, plus totals them up. The meal plan is based on a daily intake of 1500 to 2,000 calories (give or take 100 calories) and an approximate Macro ratio of 70% to 80% fat, 10% to 20% protein, and 5% to 10% carbohydrates.

4-Week Basic Meal Plan

Week 1 Meal Plan				
Day	Breakfast	Lunch	Dinner	Snack/Dessert	Calories/Macros
1	Strawberry Cow Smoothie 301 cal 28.6 g fat 2.8 g protein 9 g carbs	Cilantro Lime Shrimp and Avocado Salad 529 cal 35.6 g fat 26 g protein 5 g carbs	Spinach Stuffed Cod 407 cal 13.7 g fat 65.6 g protein 1 g carbs	Seed Crackers & Guacamole 280 cal 24 g fat 8 g protein 3 g carbs	Calories: 1517 Fat: 101.9 g Protein: 82.4 g Net Carbs: 18 g

2	Coconut Macadamia Smoothie Bowl 362 cal 33.5 g fat 3.2 g protein 8 g carbs	Cream of Leek Soup with Seed Crackers 175 cal 14.5 g fat 4.3 g protein 3 g carbs	Roast Chicken (1 serving) with Butter Tossed Asparagus 280 cal 30 g fat 14 g protein 3 g carbs	Almond Butter Fat Bombs (2) 378 cal 38.2 g fat 6.4 g protein 2.8 g carbs	Calories: 1195 Fat: 116.2 g Protein: 31.1 g Net Carbs: 18.2 g
3	Almond Butter Smoothie 483 cal 34.6 g fat 5.5 g protein 4 g carbs	Chicken Salad 367 cal 25 g fat 34 g protein 2 g carbs	Beef Fajita Bowl 360 cal 12 g fat 48 g protein 11 g carbs	Nordic Seed Bread 369 cal 31.5 g fat 10 g protein 5 g carbs	Calories: 1579 Fat: 103.1 g Protein: 85.5 g Net Carbs: 22 g
4	Keto Eggs Benedict with Quick Hollandaise Sauce 757 cal 68 g fat 35 g protein 5 g carbs	Asian Salad with Asian Nut Dressing 579 cal 55.4 g fat 5 g protein 9 g carbs	Chicken Avocado Pesto Pasta 440 cal 40 g fat 36 g protein 3 g carbs	Almond Butter Fat Bomb 189 cal 19.1 g fat 3.2 g protein 1.4 g carbs	Calories: 1965 Fat: 182.5 g Protein: 79.2 g Net Carbs: 18.4 g
5	Beef Frittata (from leftover Beef Fajita Bowl) 584 cal 42 g fat 39 g protein 9.7 g carbs	Avocado and Chicken Salad 663 cal 55 g fat 28 g protein 6 g carbs	Pork Chops with Green Bean Fries 481 cal 37 g fat 39 g protein 2 g carbs	Celery and Almond Butter 230 cal 18 g fat 8 g protein 4 g carbs	Calories: 1958 Fat: 152 g Protein: 114 g Net Carbs: 21.7 g

6	Avocado Pesto Eggs

404 cal

37 g fat

4 g protein

4.6 g carbs | Pork Chopped Salad

681 cal

57.9 g fat

29 g protein

9 g carbs | Greek Lamb Burger

542 cal

40 g fat

36 g protein

5 g carbs | Chocolate Smoothie

575 cal

44 g fat

34 g protein

3 g carbs | Calories: 2202

Fat: 178.9 g

Protein: 103 g

Net Carbs: 21.6 g |
| 7 | Vanilla Smoothie

669 cal

70.8 g fat

5.5 g protein

4 g carbs | Lettuce Wrapped Lamb Burgers

513 cal

37 g fat

34 g protein

9 g carbs | Thai Chicken Coconut Red Curry

310 cal

26 g fat

14 g protein

7 g carbs | Raspberry Chia Pudding

642 cal

50 g fat

15.9 g protein

8 g carbs | Calories: 2134

Fat: 183.8 g

Protein: 69.4 g

Net Carbs: 28 g |

Day	Breakfast	Lunch	Dinner	Snack/Dessert	Calories/Macros
			Week 2 Meal Plan		
8	2 Eggs (any style) and 2 strips of Bacon with Bulletproof Coffee 585 cal 56.5 g fat 21 g protein 3 g carbs	Cream of Mushroom Soup 222 cal 15.6 g fat 7.8 g protein 11 g carbs	Lamb Chops with Buttery Mustard Sauce 429 cal 27 g fat 25 g protein 9 g carbs	Seed Crackers & Guacamole 280 cal 24 g fat 8 g protein 3 g carbs	Calories: 1516 Fat: 123.1 g Protein: 61.8 g Net Carbs: 26 g
9	Pink Power Smoothie 310 cal 29.9 g fat 3.8 g protein 9 g carbs	Lemon Thyme Salmon Salad with Lemon Thyme Vinaigrette 402 cal 21.1 g fat 41.7 g protein 9.1 g carbs	Indian Butter Chicken with Roasted Cauliflower 592 cal 52 g fat 24 g protein 6 g carbs	Nordic Seed Bread 369 cal 31.5 g fat 10 g protein 5 g carbs	Calories: 1673 Fat: 134.5 g Protein: 79.5 g Net Carbs: 29.1g
10	Breakfast Sausages 326 cal 28 g fat 19 g protein 0 g carbs	Creamy Tomato Soup 135 cal 10.1 g fat 2.5 g protein 6 g carbs	Goat Cheese Stuffed Chicken Breasts 646 cal 44.5 g fat 55.9 g protein 3 g carbs	Raspberry Chocolate Fudge 74 cal 8.1 g fat 0.6 g protein 0.9 g carbs	Calories: 1181 Fat: 90.7 g Protein: 78 g Net Carbs: 9.9 g

11	Mushroom and Bacon Skillet 591 cal 47.7 g fat 36 g protein 3 g carbs	Italian Chopped Salad 469 cal 44 g fat 14 g protein 4 g carbs	Beef Stuffed Tomatoes 350 cal 15.5 g fat 36 g protein 5 g carbs	Mediterranean Fat Bomb 155 cal 15 g fat 3 g protein 1.2 g carbs	Calories: 1565 Fat: 122.2 g Protein: 89 g Net Carbs: 13.2 g
12	Coconut Macadamia Smoothie Bowl 362 cal 33.5 g fat 3.2 g protein 8 g carbs	Baja Style Halibut Salad 740 cal 40 g fat 95 g protein 7 g carbs	Baked Eggs with Kale and Tomato 187 cal 15.3 g fat 9 g protein 3 g carbs	Vanilla Smoothie 669 cal 70.8 g fat 5.5 g protein 4 g carbs	Calories: 1958 Fat: 159.6 g Protein: 112.7 g Net Carbs: 22 g
13	Bell Pepper Eggs 298 cal 26.2 g fat 11.9 g protein 4 g carbs	Kale Salad 322 cal 30.9 g fat 2.9 g protein 9 g carbs	Fish Tacos 740 cal 40 g fat 95 g protein 7 g carbs	Salted Macadamias 224 cal 22 g fat 3 g protein 1 g carbs	Calories: 1584 Fat: 119.1 g Protein: 112.8 g Net Carbs: 21 g
14	Breakfast Beef Skillet 705 cal 58.7 g fat 36.4 g protein 4 g carbs	Nicoise Salad 273 cal 20 g fat 23 g protein 2 g carbs	Jerk Chicken 524 cal 33.9 g fat 44 g protein 5 g carbs	Cheesy Fondue 376 cal 32 g fat 19.5 g protein 4.4 g carbs	Calories: 1878 Fat: 144.6 g Protein: 122.9 g Net Carbs: 15.4 g

		Week 3 Meal Plan			
Day	Breakfast	Lunch	Dinner	Snack/Dessert	Calories/Macros
15	Caprese Omelet 393 cal 35.9 g fat 11.3 g protein 6 g carbs	Leftover Jerk Chicken 524 cal 33.9 g fat 44 g protein 5 g carbs	Beef Kababs 219 cal 15.7 g fat 16 g protein 2 g carbs	Strawberry Chia Pudding Popsicles 277 cal 24.9 g fat 5 g protein 3 g carbs	Calories: 1413 Fat: 110.4 g Protein: 76.3 g Net Carbs: 16 g
16	Cream Cheese and Herb Pancakes with Smoked Salmon and Dill 417 cal 35.8 g fat 20 g protein 3 g carbs	Steak and Avocado Salad with Cilantro Lime Dressing 663 cal 44 g fat 50 g protein 7 g carbs	Thai Chicken Coconut Red Curry 310 cal 26 g fat 14 g protein 7 g carbs	Golden Milk Smoothie 460 cal 25.3 g fat 1.7 g protein 1.4 g carbs	Calories: 1850 Fat: 131.1 g Protein: 85.7 g Net Carbs: 18.4 g
17	Cuban Frittata 282 cal 21.6 g fat 17.7 g protein 3 g carbs	Avocado and Chicken Salad 663 cal 55 g fat 28 g protein 6 g carbs	Beef Stew 450 cal 30.4 g fat 35 g protein 4.5 g carbs	Nordic Seed Bread 369 cal 31.5 g fat 10 g protein 5 g carbs	Calories: 1764 Fat: 138.5 g Protein: 90.7 g Net Carbs: 18.5 g

18	Nordic Seed Bread Breakfast Sandwich 434 cal 40 g fat 32 g protein 4 g carbs	Warm Zucchini and Goat Cheese Salad 395 cal 35.5 g fat 14.8 g protein 6 g carbs	Parmesan Crusted Halibut 266 cal 14.8 g fat 30 g protein 1.2 g carbs	Almond Butter Cookies 98 cal 10 g fat 4 g protein 1.4 g carbs	Calories: 1193 Fat: 115.5 g Protein: 80.8 g Net Carbs: 12.6 g
19	Scotch Eggs 442 cal 46 g fat 25 g protein 0 g carbs	Creamy Cauliflower and Seafood Chowder 540 cal 52 g fat 28 g protein 7 g carbs	Chicken Kababs 270 cal 17.2 g fat 25 g protein 2 g carbs	Tahini Sauce with Veggies 555 cal 58.5 g fat 4 g protein 8 g carbs	Calories: 1807 Fat: 173.7 g Protein: 82 g Net Carbs: 17 g
20	Strawberry Cow Smoothie 301 cal 28.6 g fat 2.8 g protein 9 g carbs	Scallop and Mushroom Salad with Goat Cheese Vinaigrette 498 cal 38.8 g fat 32.7 g protein 4.4 g carbs	Beef Vindaloo 436 cal 30.4 g fat 35 g protein 3.5 g carbs	Seed Crackers and Guacamole 280 cal 24 g fat 8 g protein 3 g carbs	Calories: 1515 Fat: 121.8 g Protein: 78.5 g Net Carbs: 19.9 g
21	Cream Cheese and Lox Omelet 731 cal 61.9 g fat 40.9 g protein 3.5 g carbs	Cream of Mushroom Soup 222 cal 15.6 g fat 7.8 g protein 11 g carbs	Chicken Avocado Pesto Pasta 440 cal 40 g fat 36 g protein 3 g carbs	Raspberry Chia Pudding 642 cal 50 g fat 15.9 g protein 8 g carbs	Calories: 2035 Fat: 167.5 g Protein: 100.6 g Net Carbs: 25.5 g

		Week 4 Meal Plan			
Day	Breakfast	Lunch	Dinner	Snack/Dessert	Calories/Macros
22	2 Eggs (any style), 2 Strips of Bacon, and Bulletproof Coffee 585 cal 56.5 g fat 21 g protein 3 g carbs	Chicken Kale Wrap 415 cal 32.1 g fat 26.3 g protein 5.3 g carbs	Thai Coconut Cod 482 cal 34 g fat 42.5 g protein 5 g carbs	Almond Butter Fat Bomb 189 cal 19.1 g fat 3.2 g protein 1.4 g carbs	Calories: 1671 Fat: 141.7 g Protein: 93 g Net Carbs: 14.7 g
23	Almond Butter Smoothie 300 cal 31 g fat 7 g protein 4 g carbs	Thai Coconut Cod Lettuce Wraps 592 cal 46 g fat 35 g protein 6 g carbs	Cheese Stuffed Burgers 681 cal 44.7 g fat 63.1 g protein 3.7 g carbs	Green Bean Fries 113 cal 6 g fat 9 g protein 2 g carbs	Calories: 1686 Fat: 127.7 g Protein: 114.1 g Net Carbs: 15.7 g
24	Mushroom and Goat Cheese Omelet 818 cal 74.1 g fat 35.8 g protein 3 g carbs	Kale Salad 322 cal 30.9 g fat 2.9 g protein 9 g carbs	Keto Chinese Beef and Broccoli 273 cal 17 g fat 24 g protein 3 g carbs	Chocolate Smoothie 575 cal 44 g fat 34 g protein 3 g carbs	Calories: 1988 Fat: 166 g Protein: 96.7 g Net Carbs: 18 g

25	Avocado Breakfast Sandwich 698 cal 61 g fat 24.1 g protein 5.5 g carbs	Creamy Tomato Soup 135 cal 10.1 g fat 2.5 g protein 6 g carbs	Sea Bass with Prosciutto and Herbs 586 cal 16.2 g fat 40 g protein 6 g carbs	Almond Butter Cookies 98 cal 10 g fat 4 g protein 1.4 g carbs	Calories: 1517 Fat: 97.3 g Protein: 70.6 g Net Carbs: 18.9 g
26	Pink Power Smoothie 310 cal 29.9 g fat 3.8 g protein 9 g carbs	Steak and Avocado Salad 663 cal 44 g fat 50 g protein 7 g carbs	Goat Cheese Stuffed Chicken Breasts 646 cal 44.5 g fat 55.9 g protein 3 g carbs	Celery and Almond Butter 230 cal 18 g fat 8 g protein 4 g carbs	Calories: 1849 Fat: 136.4 g Protein: 117.7 g Net Carbs: 23 g
27	Bell Pepper Eggs 298 cal 26.2 g fat 11.9 g protein 4 g carbs	Leftover Goat Cheese Chicken Breasts 646 cal 44.5 g fat 55.9 g protein 3 g carbs	Steak and Avocado Taco Cups 650 cal 53 g fat 40 g protein 6 g carbs	Veggies with Spicy Mayo 90 cal 10 g fat 0 g protein 0 g carbs	Calories: 1684 Fat: 133.7 g Protein: 107.8 g Net Carbs: 13 g
28	Chocolate Smoothie 575 cal 44 g fat 34 g protein 3 g carbs	Cream of Leek Soup 175 cal 14.5 g fat 4.3 g protein 3 g carbs	Chicken Avocado Pesto Pasta 440 cal 40 g fat 36 g protein 3 g carbs	Nordic Seed Bread 369 cal 31.5 g fat 10 g protein 5 g carbs	Calories: 1559 Fat: 130 g Protein: 84.3 g Net Carbs: 14 g

Busy households will definitely appreciate the 30 minute fast meal plan. This is excellent for Keto dieters with a family, a demanding job, or when it's summer and too hot to cook in the kitchen!

4-Week Fast Meal Plan With 30-Minute Meals

Week 1 Meal Plan					
Day	Breakfast	Lunch	Dinner	Snack/Dessert	Calories/Macros
1	Strawberry Cow Smoothie 301 cal 28.6 g fat 2.8 g protein 9 g carbs	Cilantro Lime Shrimp and Avocado Salad 529 cal 35.6 g fat 26 g protein 5 g carbs	Beef Stuffed Tomatoes 350 cal 15.5 g fat 36 g protein 5 g carbs	Almond Butter Fat Bomb 189 cal 19.1 g fat 3.2 g protein 1.4 g carbs	Calories: 1369 Fat: 98.8 g Protein: 68 g Net Carbs: 20.4 g
2	Coconut Macadamia Smoothie Bowl 362 cal 33.5 g fat 3.2 g protein 8 g carbs	Cream of Mushroom Soup 222 cal 15.6 g fat 7.8 g protein 11 g carbs	Beef Fajita Bowl 360 cal 12 g fat 48 g protein 11 g carbs	Mediterranean Fat Bomb 155 cal 15 g fat 3 g protein 1.2 g carbs	Calories: 1099 Fat: 76.1 g Protein: 62 g Net Carbs: 29 g
3	Almond Butter Smoothie 300 cal 31 g fat 7 g protein 4 g carbs	Beef Fajita Lettuce Wraps 513 cal 37 g fat 34 g protein 9 g carbs	Chicken Avocado Pesto Pasta 440 cal 40 g fat 36 g protein 3 g carbs	Veggies and Green Tahini 43 cal 3.9 g fat 0.7 g protein 0.3 g carbs	Calories: 1296 Fat: 111.9 g Protein: 77.7 g Net Carbs: 16.3 g

4	Beef Frittata 584 cal 42 g fat 39 g protein 9.7 g carbs	Asian Salad with Asian Nut Dressing 579 cal 55.4 g fat 5 g protein 9 g carbs	Greek Lamb Burger 542 cal 40 g fat 36 g protein 5 g carbs	Chocolate Smoothie 575 cal 44 g fat 34 g protein 3 g carbs	Calories: 2280 Fat: 181.4 g Protein: 114 g Net Carbs: 26.7 g
5	Vanilla Smoothie 669 cal 70.8 g fat 5.5 g protein 4 g carbs	Avocado and Chicken Salad 663 cal 55 g fat 28 g protein 6 g carbs	Cod Bruschetta 341 cal 18.2 g fat 28.4 g protein 3.5 g carbs	Raspberry Chia Pudding 642 cal 50 g fat 15.9 g protein 8 g carbs	Calories: 2315 Fat: 194 g Protein: 77.8 g Net Carbs: 21.5 g
6	2 Eggs (any style) and 2 Strips of Bacon with Bulletproof Coffee 585 cal 56.5 g fat 21 g protein 3 g carbs	Lettuce Wrapped Lamb Burgers 513 cal 37 g fat 34 g protein 9 g carbs	Thai Chicken Coconut Red Curry 310 cal 26 g fat 14 g protein 7 g carbs	Chocolate Smoothie 575 cal 44 g fat 34 g protein 3 g carbs	Calories: 1983 Fat: 163.5 g Protein: 103 g Net Carbs: 22 g
7	Pink Power Smoothie 310 cal 29.9 g fat 3.8 g protein 9 g carbs	Lemon Thyme Salmon Salad with Lemon Thyme Vinaigrette 402 cal 21.1 g fat 41.7 g protein 9.1 g carbs	Mushroom and Bacon Skillet 591 cal 47.7 g fat 36 g protein 3 g carbs	Celery and Almond Butter 230 cal 18 g fat 8 g protein 4 g carbs	Calories: 1533 Fat: 116.7 g Protein: 89.5 g Net Carbs: 25.1 g

		Week 2 Meal Plan			
Day	Breakfast	Lunch	Dinner	Snack/Dessert	Calories/Macros
8	Caprese Omelet 393 cal 35.9 g fat 11.3 g protein 6 g carbs	Nicoise Salad 273 cal 20 g fat 23 g protein 2 g carbs	Beef Stuffed Tomatoes 350 cal 15.5 g fat 36 g protein 5 g carbs	Raspberry Chocolate Fudge 74 cal 8.1 g fat 0.6 g protein 0.9 g carbs	Calories: 1090 Fat: 79.5 g Protein: 70.9 g Net Carbs: 13.9 g
9	Breakfast Sausages 326 cal 28 g fat 19 g protein 0 g carbs	Baja Style Halibut Salad 740 cal 40 g fat 95 g protein 7 g carbs	Keto Chinese Beef and Broccoli 273 cal 17 g fat 24 g protein 3 g carbs	Golden Milk Smoothie 460 cal 25.3 g fat 1.7 g protein 1.4 g carbs	Calories: 1799 Fat: 110.3 g Protein: 109.7 g Net Carbs: 11.4 g
10	Cream Cheese and Herb Pancakes with Smoked Salmon and Dill 417 cal 35.8 g fat 20 g protein 3 g carbs	Egg Salad 242 cal 18.6 g fat 11.4 g protein 8 g carbs	Fish Tacos 740 cal 40 g fat 95 g protein 7 g carbs	Salted Macadamias 224 cal 22 g fat 3 g protein 1 g carbs	Calories: 1623 Fat: 116.4 g Protein: 99.4 g Net Carbs: 19 g

11	Bell Pepper Eggs 298 cal 26.2 g fat 11.9 g protein 4 g carbs	Kale Salad 322 cal 30.9 g fat 2.9 g protein 9 g carbs	Lamb Chops with Buttery Mustard Sauce 429 cal 27 g fat 25 g protein 9 g carbs	Vanilla Smoothie 669 cal 70.8 g fat 5.5 g protein 4 g carbs	Calories: 1718 Fat: 154.9 g Protein: 45.3 g Net Carbs: 26 g
12	Lemon Cream Pancakes 351 cal 30.3 g fat 6.7 g protein 4 g carbs	Leftover Lamb Chops 429 cal 27 g fat 25 g protein 9 g carbs	Steak and Avocado Salad 663 cal 44 g fat 50 g protein 7 g carbs	Raspberry Chia Pudding 642 cal 50 g fat 15.9 g protein 8 g carbs	Calories: 2085 Fat: 151.3 g Protein: 97.6 g Net Carbs: 28 g
13	Coconut Macadamia Smoothie Bowl 362 cal 33.5 g fat 3.2 g protein 8 g carbs	Cream of Mushroom Soup 222 cal 15.6 g fat 7.8 g protein 11 g carbs	Steak and Avocado Taco Cups 650 cal 53 g fat 40 g protein 6 g carbs	Chocolate Smoothie 575 cal 44 g fat 34 g protein 3 g carbs	Calories: 1809 Fat: 146.1 g Protein: 85 g Net Carbs: 28 g
14	Avocado Breakfast Sandwich 698 cal 61 g fat 24.1 g protein 5.5 g carbs	Italian Chopped Salad 469 cal 44 g fat 14 g protein 4 g carbs	Thai Coconut Cod 482 cal 34 g fat 42.5 g protein 5 g carbs	Almond Butter Fat Bomb 189 cal 19.1 g fat 3.2 g protein 1.4 g carbs	Calories: 1838 Fat: 158.1 g Protein: 83.8 g Net Carbs: 15.9 g

		Week 3 Meal Plan			
Day	Breakfast	Lunch	Dinner	Snack/Dessert	Calories/Macros
15	Keto Breakfast Bowl 489 cal 35 g fat 29 g protein 4 g carbs	Thai Coconut Cod Lettuce Wraps 592 cal 46 g fat 35 g protein 6 g carbs	Chicken Avocado Pesto Pasta 440 cal 40 g fat 36 g protein 3 g carbs	Almond Butter Smoothie 300 cal 31 g fat 7 g protein 4 g carbs	Calories: 1821 Fat: 152 g Protein: 107 g Net Carbs: 17 g
16	Avocado Pesto Eggs 404 cal 37 g fat 4 g protein 4.6 g carbs	Lemon Thyme Salmon Salad with Lemon Thyme Vinaigrette 402 cal 21.1 g fat 41.7 g protein 9.1 g carbs	Beef Fajita Bowl 360 cal 12 g fat 48 g protein 11 g carbs	Almond Butter Cookies 98 cal 10 g fat 4 g protein 1.4 g carbs	Calories: 1264 Fat: 97.7 g Protein: 80.1 g Net Carbs: 26.1 g
17	Scotch Eggs 442 cal 46 g fat 25 g protein 0 g carbs	Beef Fajita Lettuce Wraps 513 cal 37 g fat 34 g protein 9 g carbs	Thai Chicken Coconut Red Curry 310 cal 26 g fat 14 g protein 7 g carbs	Strawberry Cow Smoothie 301 cal 28.6 g fat 2.8 g protein 9 g carbs	Calories: 1566 Fat: 137.6 g Protein: 75.8 g Net Carbs: 25 g

18	Coconut Porridge 400 cal 39 g fat 13 g protein 5 g carbs	Kale Salad 322 cal 30.9 g fat 2.9 g protein 9 g carbs	Mushroom and Goat Cheese Omelet 818 cal 74.1 g fat 35.8 g protein 3 g carbs	Chocolate Smoothie 575 cal 44 g fat 34 g protein 3 g carbs	Calories: 2115 Fat: 188 g Protein: 85.7 g Net Carbs: 20 g
19	Baked Eggs with Kale and Tomato 187 cal 15.3 g fat 9 g protein 3 g carbs	Italian Chopped Salad 469 cal 44 g fat 14 g protein 4 g carbs	Crab Stuffed Avocado 319 cal 25.7 g fat 9.4 g protein 6 g carbs	Mediterranean Fat Bomb 155 cal 15 g fat 3 g protein 1.2 g carbs	Calories: 1130 Fat: 100 g Protein: 35.4 g Net Carbs: 14.2 g
20	Cuban Frittata 282 cal 21.6 g fat 17.7 g protein 3 g carbs	Nicoise Salad 273 cal 20 g fat 23 g protein 2 g carbs	Greek Lamb Burger 542 cal 40 g fat 36 g protein 5 g carbs	Veggies with Tahini Sauce 555 cal 58.5 g fat 4 g protein 8 g carbs	Calories: 1652 Fat: 140.1 g Protein: 80.7 g Net Carbs: 18 g
21	Vanilla Smoothie 669 cal 70.8 g fat 5.5 g protein 4 g carbs	Lettuce Wrapped Lamb Burger 513 cal 37 g fat 34 g protein 9 g carbs	Mushroom and Bacon Skillet 591 cal 47.7 g fat 36 g protein 3 g carbs	Green Bean Fries 113 cal 6 g fat 9 g protein 2 g carbs	Calories: 1886 Fat: 161.5 g Protein: 84.5 g Net Carbs: 18 g

Day	Breakfast	Lunch	Dinner	Snack/Dessert	Calories/Macros
		Week 4 Meal Plan			
22	2 Eggs (any style), 2 strips of Bacon, and Bulletproof Coffee 585 cal 56.5 g fat 21 g protein 3 g carbs	Green Salad with Green Goddess Dressing 316 cal 32 g fat 2 g protein 2 g carbs	Thai Coconut Cod 482 cal 34 g fat 42.5 g protein 5 g carbs	Golden Milk Smoothie 460 cal 25.3 g fat 1.7 g protein 1.4 g carbs	Calories: 1843 Fat: 147.8 g Protein: 67.2 g Net Carbs: 11.4 g
23	Caprese Omelet 393 cal 35.9 g fat 11.3 g protein 6 g carbs	Thai Coconut Cod Lettuce Wraps 482 cal 34 g fat 42.5 g protein 5 g carbs	Beef Stuffed Tomatoes 350 cal 15.5 g fat 36 g protein 5 g carbs	Raspberry Chocolate Fudge 74 cal 8.1 g fat 0.6 g protein 0.9 g carbs	Calories: 1299 Fat: 106.5 g Protein: 90.4 g Net Carbs: 16.9 g
24	Baked Eggs with Kale and Tomato 187 cal 15.3 g fat 9 g protein 3 g carbs	Cilantro Lime Shrimp and Avocado Salad 529 cal 35.6 g fat 26 g protein 5 g carbs	Thai Chicken Coconut Red Curry 310 cal 26 g fat 14 g protein 7 g carbs	Celery and Almond Butter 230 cal 18 g fat 8 g protein 4 g carbs	Calories: 1256 Fat: 94.9 g Protein: 57 g Net Carbs: 19 g

25	Coconut Porridge 400 cal 39 g fat 13 g protein 5 g carbs	Avocado and Chicken Salad 663 cal 55 g fat 28 g protein 6 g carbs	Cod Bruschetta 341 cal 18.2 g fat 28.4 g protein 3.5 g carbs	Chocolate Smoothie 575 cal 44 g fat 34 g protein 3 g carbs	Calories: 1979 Fat: 101.75 g Protein: 83.4 g Net Carbs: 17.5 g
26	Scotch Eggs 442 cal 46 g fat 25 g protein 0 g carbs	Italian Chopped Salad 469 cal 44 g fat 14 g protein 4 g carbs	Keto Chinese Beef and Broccoli 273 cal 17 g fat 24 g protein 3 g carbs	Almond Butter Fat Bomb 189 cal 19.1 g fat 3.2 g protein 1.4 g carbs	Calories: 1373 Fat: 126.1 g Protein: 66.2 g Net Carbs: 8.4 g
27	Almond Butter Smoothie 300 cal 31 g fat 7 g protein 4 g carbs	Crab Stuffed Cucumbers 179 cal 17.4 g fat 3.1 g protein 3 g carbs	Chicken Avocado Pesto Pasta 440 cal 40 g fat 36 g protein 3 g carbs	Salted Macadamias 224 cal 22 g fat 3 g protein 1 g carbs	Calories: 1143 Fat: 110.4 g Protein: 49.1 g Net Carbs: 11 g
28	Lemon Cream Pancakes 351 cal 30.3 g fat 6.7 g protein 4 g carbs	Kale Salad 322 cal 30.9 g fat 2.9 g protein 9 g carbs	Lamb Chops with Buttery Mustard Sauce 429 cal 27 g fat 25 g protein 9 g carbs	Strawberry Cow Smoothie 301 cal 28.6 g fat 2.8 g protein 9 g carbs	Calories: 1403 Fat: 116.8 g Protein: 37.4 g Net Carbs: 29 g

Chapter 8:
K For Keto Recipes

After looking at the meal plans in the previous chapter, I hope you're excited to get cooking! In this chapter, you'll see the following seven sections:

- Breakfast
- Soups and Salads
- Pork and Poultry
- Beef and Lamb
- Seafood
- Desserts and Drinks
- Snacks and Sides

There are over 100 recipes here to inspire you. Think of these as launch points for your brand new Ketogenic adventure. Have fun with them, experiment with them, and make them your own.

Bon Appetit!

Breakfast

Keto Breakfast Bowl

Protein and flavor packed, this breakfast bowl will keep you full and satisfied for hours! It's really good for you and really delicious, too.

Serving: 1

Serving Size: whole recipe

Prep Time: 5 minutes

Cook Time: 5 minutes

Ingredients

    2 eggs

    50 g smoked salmon

    1/2 avocado

    2 cups kale

    1 teaspoon olive oil

    1 teaspoon coconut oil

Instructions

Start by chopping and washing the kale. Heat up a pan on medium heat with a little bit of olive oil and add the kale for about 5 minutes. While the kale is sautéing prepare the eggs the way you like them (scrambled, sunny side up, fried, etc..). Lastly slice up half an avocado and measure out 50 grams of smoked salmon. Once everything is ready combine in a wide bowl and enjoy.

Nutrition: 489 calories, 35g fat, 29g protein, 4g net carbs

Coconut Porridge

This porridge has a great consistency, and comes together very easily.

Serving: 2

Serving Size: 1 cup

Prep Time: 5 minutes

Cook Time: 10 minutes

Ingredients

¼ cup coconut flour

¼ cup ground flax

1 egg, beaten

1 ½ cups water

1 Tablespoon butter

2 Tablespoons heavy cream

1 Tablespoon Stevia

Instructions

Mix together the water, coconut flour and flax in a medium sized saucepan. Turn the heat on to high, and bring to a boil. Reduce heat to low, and simmer until it begins to thicken, about 5 minutes. Beat in the egg until smooth. Add in the butter, cream and sweetener right away, and stir until smooth.

Nutrition: 400 calories, 39 g fat, 13 g protein, 5 g net carbs

Coconut Macadamia Smoothie Bowl

This satisfying smoothie is a great snack or breakfast option! The creamy, crunchy macadamia nuts go really well with the smooth coconut milk, giving this bowl lots of great texture and flavor!

Serving: 1

Serving Size: whole recipe

Prep Time: 10 minutes

Cook Time: 0 minutes

Ingredients

> ½ cup coconut milk
>
> 1 teaspoon Stevia
>
> ¼ cup macadamia nuts
>
> 1 Tablespoon coconut flakes
>
> ¼ teaspoon salt
>
> 1 teaspoon cinnamon

Instructions

Whisk together the coconut cream, coconut milk, Stevia, salt and cinnamon. Spoon the mixture into a bowl, and top with the macadamia nuts and coconut flakes. Serve immediately, or keep in the fridge for up to a day.

> Nutrition: 362 calories, 33.5 g fat, 3.2 g protein, 8g net carbs

Caprese Omelet

Try this yummy omelet with a side of hash browns or sausage! This is a basic omelet recipe you can dress up with all kinds of Keto friendly ingredients: spinach and feta, mushroom and sausage, bacon and onion, Mexican salsa, etc. Have fun in the kitchen.

Serving: 2

Serving Size: half recipe

Prep Time: 5 minutes

Cook Time: 10 minutes

Ingredients

> 3 eggs
>
> ¼ cup butter
>
> ¼ cup heavy cream
>
> ¼ cup mozzarella, shredded
>
> 2 Tablespoons parmesan
>
> 4 cherry tomatoes, sliced in half
>
> Handful basil, chopped roughly

Instructions

Whisk together the eggs and cream. Season with salt and pepper. Preheat a medium pan over medium high heat, and melt the butter. Pour in the egg mixture, and let cook 3-4 minutes. Gently flip, cooking the other side. Top with the cheeses, tomato and basil, and gently fold. Cook another 3-4 minutes. Cut in half. Serve immediately.

Nutrition: 393 calories, 35.9 g fat, 11.3 g protein, 6 g net carbs

Mushroom and Goat Cheese Omelet

Such a yummy classic French recipe! You can add some sliced shallots and a sprinkle of light shredded cheddar if you have it, too.

Serving: 2

Serving Size: Half Omelet

Prep Time: 5 minutes

Cook Time:10 minutes

Ingredients

> 6 eggs
>
> ½ cup mushrooms, sliced
>
> ¼ lb goat cheese
>
> 2 Tablespoons butter
>
> 1 Tablespoon olive oil
>
> 1 cup heavy cream

Instructions

Beat together the eggs and cream. Preheat a medium pan over medium heat. Drizzle in the oil and melt in the butter. Sauté the mushrooms with a pinch of salt until soft, about 1 minute. Pour in the egg mixture and cook for 3-5 minutes, until the bottom has set. Flip, and cook the other side. Lay the goat cheese on top, and fold the omelet. Serve warm.

> Nutrition: 818 calories, 74.1 g fat,35.8 g protein, 3 g net carbs

Cream Cheese and Lox Omelet

Lox- also known by its more official term Smoked Salmon- is a high fat, high flavor breakfast favorite! This omelet combines creamy cream cheese with smoked salmon and dill for a fun, fast breakfast option!

Serving: 2

Serving Size: ½ omelet

Prep Time: 5 minutes

Cook Time: 10 minutes

Ingredients

> ½ lb smoked salmon, cut into ribbons
>
> 2 Tablespoons butter
>
> 6 eggs

1 cup heavy cream

¼ cup cream cheese

Handful dill, chopped

Instructions

Preheat a medium sized pan over medium heat. Drizzle in the oil and melt the butter. Mix the eggs and cream with a bit of salt, and pour the mixture into the pan. Allow the bottom to set, about 3 minutes, then flip. Cook until the other side has set, about 3 minutes longer. Spoon the cream cheese over top, followed by the smoked salmon and dill. Fold the omelet in half. Cook until the cheese starts to melt and ooze, about 3 minutes. Serve warm.

Nutrition: 731 calories, 61.9 g fat, 40.9 g protein, 3.5 g net carbs

Breakfast Sausage

The problem with store bought sausage is that it's normally full of sugar, carb-laden fillers, and other Keto no nos! Luckily, making your own sausage is a snap! These sausages are delicious, full of great fat, and can be made in batches and kept in the fridge for up to a week, or the freezer for up to 4 months.

Serving: 4

Serving Size: 2 Patties

Prep Time: 5 minutes

Cook Time: 10 minutes

Ingredients

1 lb ground pork

1 Tablespoon Italian herbs

1/2 Tablespoon garlic powder

1/2 Tablespoon onion powder

2 teaspoons fennel

1/2 teaspoon salt

1/2 teaspoon pepper

Instructions

In a large bowl combine the ground pork with all of the seasonings. Mix the seasoning into the meat as well as possible and then form 8 patties. Heat a pan on medium heat and add the coconut oil. Once the coconut oil is melted add all of the patties or if you can only fit 4 save half of the oil for the second batch. Fry the patties for 3-5 minutes on each side or until cooked through and golden brown on the outside. Serve warm, or store in an airtight container in the fridge for up to a week.

Nutrition: 326 calories, 28g fat, 19g protein, 0g net carbs

Scotch Eggs

Scotch eggs are traditionally soft-boiled eggs that have been coated in sausage and breading, and deep fried! The perfect Scotch egg is gooey in the center, and crispy on the outside with a thick coating of perfectly seasoned sausage all around! Using the base recipe for Breakfast Sausages, these eggs come together quickly and easily, and are the perfect addition to a keto friendly brunch!

Serving: 4

Serving Size: 1 egg

Prep Time: 5 minutes

Cook Time: 10 minutes

Ingredients

> 1 serving Breakfast Sausage, uncooked
>
> 4 eggs
>
> 1 cup ground pork rinds
>
> 6 cups oil, for frying

Instructions

Soft boil the eggs- In a medium sized saucepan with 1 cup of water in the bottom, boil the eggs for 4 minutes. Transfer to an ice bath, and allow to cool. Peel carefully, making sure not to break the egg. Divide the sausage meat into four portions, as you would for patties, and gently pack each portion around each egg. Next, pour the oil into a large pot and bring to a temperature of 350f on the stove, using a candy thermometer. Roll the sausage-coated eggs in the pork rinds, and fry for 2-4 minutes, until the eggs begin to float. Remove from heat, drain on a paper towel, and serve immediately.

> Nutrition: 442 calories, 46g fat, 25g protein, 0g net carbs

Baked Eggs with Kale and Tomato

This hearty skillet is the perfect thing for a chilly morning! You can substitute spinach for the kale, but make sure it's fresh.

Serving: 2

Serving Size: ½ skillet

Prep Time: 5 minutes

Cook Time: 10 minutes

Ingredients

> ½ tomato, diced
>
> ¼ cup kale, chopped
>
> 1 teaspoon garlic powder

2 Tablespoons butter

4 eggs

1 cup cream

1 teaspoon salt

1 teaspoon pepper

1 cup parmesan, shredded

Instructions

Preheat oven to 350F. Preheat a medium pan over medium heat. Melt in the butter, and sauté the kale, tomato and garlic butter together with the salt and pepper. Cook until the kale has wilted down slightly, about 3 minutes. Pour in the cream, and cook for another 3-4 minutes. Pour the mixture evenly into four ramekins. Crack an egg into each ramekin, and top with the cheese. Place the ramekins on a baking sheet, and bake for 15 minutes until the eggs are cooked and the yolks are still runny, and the cheese is bubbling. Serve warm.

Nutrition: 187 calories, 15.3 g fat, 9 g protein, 3 g net carbs

Bell Pepper Eggs

These eggs are adorable, and so easy to make! They're a variation on Toad in a Hole, where an egg is cooked in a bread ring.

Serving: 2

Serving Size: 2 eggs

Prep Time: 5 minutes

Cook Time: 15 minutes

Ingredients

1 green bell pepper, cut into ¼" rings

4 eggs

3 Tablespoons butter

Instructions

Preheat a medium pan over medium high heat. Melt in the butter, and lay the peppers down. Crack an egg into each pepper ring, and allow to cook until the whites have set and the yolk is still runny. Season with salt and pepper, and serve warm.

Nutrition: 298 calories, 26.2 g fat, 11.9 g protein, 4 g net carbs

Breakfast Beef Skillet

This hearty skillet is the perfect thing for a chilly morning!

Serving: 2

Serving Size: ½ skillet

Prep Time: 5 minutes

Cook Time: 10 minutes

Ingredients

> ½ green pepper, diced
>
> ½ tomato, diced
>
> ¼ red onion, diced
>
> ¼ lb ground beef
>
> 2 Tablespoons butter
>
> 1 Tablespoon olive oil
>
> 1 teaspoon ground cumin
>
> 1 teaspoon salt
>
> 4 eggs

Instructions

Preheat a medium sized pan over medium heat. Drizzle in the oil and melt in the butter. Add in the veggies, and sauté for 2 minutes. Add the beef and cumin, along with the salt, and cook until the beef is done, about 3-4 minutes. Crack in the eggs, and cook until the whites have set and the yolks are still runny, about 3 minutes. Serve warm.

> Nutrition:705 calories, 58.7 g fat,36.4 g protein, 4 g net carbs

Mushroom and Bacon Skillet

Sautéing mushrooms and yummy bacon in a skillet with an egg packs in the protein and gives you a fully tummy for the rest of your day. Also makes a super easy dinner.

Serving: 1

Serving Size: whole recipe

Prep Time: 10 minutes

Cook Time: 10 minutes

Ingredients

> 1 cup mushrooms, sliced
>
> 4 slices bacon, diced
>
> 1 teaspoon salt
>
> 1 egg
>
> 1 Tablespoon butter

Instructions

Melt the butter into a skillet over medium high heat. Add in the mushrooms and bacon, and sauté until done- about 5 minutes. Crack in the egg, mixing well. Season with salt and pepper.

Nutrition: 591 calories, 47.7 g fat, 36 g protein, 3 g net carbs

Nordic Seed Bread Breakfast Sandwich

When you have leftover Nordic Seed Bread, then combine it with the following ingredients to make your own breakfast sandwich, excellent for busy weekday mornings!

Serving: 1

Serving Size: whole recipe

Prep Time: 5 minutes

Cook Time: 5 minutes

Ingredients

> 1 egg, beaten
>
> 1 teaspoon mayonnaise
>
> 1 teaspoon mustard
>
> 1 small handful arugula
>
> 1 piece Nordic Seed Bread, cut in half

Instructions

Beat the egg in a small bowl, and cover. Microwave on high for 40 seconds, until fully cooked. Spread the mustard and mayo onto each slice of the seed bread. Sandwich together with the egg and arugula. Serve immediately.

Nutrition: 434 calories, 40 g fat, 32 g protein, 4g net carbs

Keto Eggs Benedict

Nordic seed bread is a great alternative to toast, making this classic recipe Keto friendly! Make the hollandaise in advance, and keep it in an airtight container in the fridge for up to four days for an easy weekday breakfast. To reheat the hollandaise, simply microwave on low for 10 second intervals until warm, or whisk in a bowl over simmering water for 10 minutes.

Serving: 1

Serving Size: whole recipe

Prep Time: 5 minutes

Cook Time: 5 minutes

Ingredients

> 1 serving Quick Hollandaise Sauce
>
> 1 egg

¼ cup water

1 serving Nordic Seed Bread (from Snacks section)

Instructions

If making the hollandaise from scratch, use the Quick Hollandaise Sauce recipe. If you already have this sauce made in the fridge, remove it from the fridge and place it in a heat-proof bowl. Bring a pot of water to a simmer, and place the bowl over top, whisking it gently for about 5 minutes until it is warm. For a quick and easy breakfast, poach the egg using the microwave technique- pour the ¼ cup of water into a microwave safe mug. Crack the egg in, and cover the mug with a plate. Microwave on high for 55 seconds. To serve, lay the seed bread onto a plate, and gently place the poached egg on top with a spoon. Spoon the hollandaise sauce over top. Serve immediately.

Nutrition: 757 calories, 68 g fat, 35 g protein, 5g net carbs

Quick Hollandaise Sauce

This sauce is the perfect topper for Keto Eggs Benedict, but can also be used at your discretion with smoked salmon and cream cheese pancakes, roasted veggies, or anything else!

Serving: 4

Serving Size: ¼ recipe

Prep Time: 5 minutes

Cook Time: 5 minutes

Ingredients

4 egg yolks

1 Tablespoon lemon juice

½ cup butter, melted

1 teaspoon cayenne

1 teaspoon salt

Instructions

In a heatproof bowl, whisk the egg yolks and lemon juice well until slightly light in color. Bring a pot of water to a simmer over medium low heat. Place the bowl with the egg yolk mixture over top of the pot of simmering water, making sure the bottom of the bowl does not touch the water. Continue to whisk quickly, and slowly whisk in the melted butter, a small bit at a time, whisking well between each addition. Whisk in the cayenne and the salt. Set aside.

Nutrition: 260 calories, 27.6 g fat, 3g protein, 1g net carb

Avocado Pesto Eggs

This fun, flavor packed recipe uses up leftover Chicken Avocado Pesto Pasta, for a fun, crispy baked egg breakfast!

Serving: 1

Serving Size:

Prep Time: 5 minutes

Cook Time: 15 minutes

Ingredients

> 1 serving Avocado Pesto Pasta

> 1 Tablespoon butter

> 1 egg

Instructions

Preheat oven to 350F. In a small pan over medium high heat, melt the butter, and toss the Avocado Pesto Pasta in, cooking for 3-4 minutes until crispy and fragrant. Transfer the crispy pasta to a small ramekin, and press in well. Crack the egg into the center of the pasta, and bake for 10 minutes. Serve immediately.

> Nutrition: 404 calories, 37 g fat, 4 g protein, 4.6 g net carbs

Cream Cheese and Herb Pancakes with Smoked Salmon and Dill

These savory pancakes are the perfect thing for brunch, breakfast or lunch. The smoked salmon, fresh dill and cream cheese compliment these pancakes beautifully!

Serving: 4

Serving Size: 2-4 pancakes (depending on size of pancake)

Prep Time: 5 minutes

Cook Time: 20 minutes

Ingredients

> 1 cup almond flour

> ½ Tablespoon dried tarragon

> ½ Tablespoon dried thyme

> 1 egg, beaten

> 1 cup heavy cream

> 1 teaspoon baking powder

> ¼ teaspoon salt

> ¼ cup butter, melted

For the sauce:

> ¼ cup cream cheese

> 1 teaspoon dried tarragon

½ teaspoon garlic powder

To top:

4 oz smoked salmon

Handful fresh dill, thyme, basil or chopped chives

Instructions

Start by making the pancakes. Whisk together the cream and egg. Mix together the almond flour, baking powder, herbs and salt. Stir in the egg mixture until smooth. Stir in the melted butter. Drizzle a bit of oil into a medium sized pan over medium heat. Spoon in a bit of the pancake batter, about 2 Tablespoons per pancake- be careful not to overcrowd the pan! Let the pancakes cook for 2-3 minutes, until the bubbles have burst. Gently flip, and cook the other side for another 1-2 minutes. Lay the finished pancakes on a plate and continue on until all the batter is used. Meanwhile, make the sauce- in a microwave safe bowl, combine all ingredients and microwave on high for 30 seconds. Beat all ingredients together until smooth. Put back into the microwave for 10 second intervals until desired consistency is reached. To serve, drizzle the cream cheese sauce over the pancakes, and top with smoked salmon and fresh herbs.

Nutrition: 417 calories, 35.8 g fat, 20 g protein, 3 g net carbs

Avocado Breakfast Sandwich

This breakfast sandwich uses an avocado bun- just like the avocado burger- to make a healthy, high fat, low carb breakfast sandwich! Beware, though! This is NOT a to-go breakfast sandwich- it's messy in a good way, but definitely one of those meals you'll want to sit down and eat with a few extra napkins!

Serving: 1

Serving Size: 1 sandwich

Prep Time: 5 minutes

Cook Time: 10 minutes

Ingredients

2 strips bacon, cooked

1 egg

1 avocado, halved

1 teaspoon sesame seeds

1 slice tomato

1 Romaine lettuce leaf

Instructions

Drizzle some oil into a small pan over medium heat. Crack in the egg, and fry to desired doneness. Using one half of the avocado as the base of your bun, top with the tomato and romaine, followed by the egg. Season with salt and pepper. Close the bun, and season with a bit more salt, then top with the sesame seeds. Serve immediately.

Nutrition: 698 calories, 61g fat, 24.1 g protein, 5.5 g net carbs

Lemon Cream Pancakes

Fluffy lemony pancakes are the perfect thing for a weekend morning! The cream cheese sauce compliments the zingy lemon perfectly.

Serving: 2

Serving Size: 1-2 pancakes

Prep Time: 5

Cook Time: 18 minutes

Ingredients

> ¼ cup almond flour
>
> 2 Tablespoons coconut flour
>
> 1 teaspoon baking powder
>
> 1 teaspoon Stevia
>
> 1 egg, beaten
>
> ¼ cup almond or coconut milk
>
> 1 teaspoon vanilla extract
>
> 1 lemon, juice and zest
>
> 1 Tablespoon butter, melted
>
> 2 Tablespoons coconut oil

For the glaze:

> 2 tbsp cream cheese
>
> 1 teaspoon powdered Stevia

Instructions

Whisk together the flours, baking powder, and Stevia. Beat together the egg, lemon juice and coconut milk with the vanilla extract. Stir in the lemon zest, and then add in the flour mixture, stirring until combined. Stir in the melted butter. Preheat a pan over medium high heat, and drizzle in the coconut oil. Spoon in the mixture, 1-2 dollops at a time. Cook 2-3 minutes, until the bubbles have burst. Gently flip the pancake over, and cook the other side for another 1-2 minutes. Next, make the glaze- In a microwave safe bowl, microwave the cream cheese on high until melted, about 1 minute. Whisk in the powdered Stevia. Drizzle the warm glaze all over the pancakes.

> Nutrition: 351 calories, 30.3 g fat, 6.7 g protein, 4 g net carbs

Beef Frittata

Frittatas are an easy, delicious way to use up leftovers! Although frittatas are typically eaten as a breakfast food, they also make a wonderful lunch or dinner as well.

Serving: 1

Serving Size: whole recipe

Prep Time: 5 minutes

Cook Time: 15 minutes

Ingredients

 1 egg, beaten

 1 Tablespoon heavy cream

 1 serving Beef Fajita Bowl

Instructions

Preheat oven to 350F. Whisk together the egg and the cream. Lay the contents of the Beef Fajita Bowl out into an oven safe ramekin, and pour the egg mixture over top. Bake for 15 minutes, until the egg has set. Serve warm.

 Nutrition: 584 calories, 42 g fat, 39 g protein, 9.7 g net carbs

Cuban Frittata

This frittata is inspired by Cuban sandwiches and is loaded with ham and cheese! Make a big batch and keep it in the fridge to use for breakfast sandwiches or on top of salads.

Serving: 4

Serving Size: ¼ frittata

Prep Time: 5 minutes

Cook Time: 25 minutes

Ingredients

 4 eggs, beaten

 1 cup heavy cream

 ½ lb ham, cooked and diced

 1 cup mozzarella, shredded

 1 tomato, diced

Instructions

Preheat oven to 350F. Whisk together the egg and the cream. Mix in the rest of the ingredients. Bake for 25 minutes, until the egg has set. Serve warm.

 Nutrition: 282 calories, 21.6 g fat, 17.7 g protein, 3 g net carbs

Soups and Salads

Creamy Tomato Soup

This soup tastes just like the classic tomato soup you enjoyed growing up, but with much more beneficial fat to keep you in ketosis! Serve with a Low Carb Grilled Cheese for an extra comforting meal!

Servings: 6

Serving Size: about 1 ½ cups

Prep Time: 10 minutes

Cook Time: 40 minutes

Ingredients:

> 2 14.5 oz cans crushed tomatoes (about 4 cups)
>
> 1 cup chicken stock
>
> ½ onion, diced
>
> 1 clove garlic, minced
>
> 2 teaspoons salt
>
> 2 teaspoons pepper
>
> 1 teaspoon nutmeg
>
> 1 teaspoon thyme
>
> 1 cup cream
>
> ¼ cup butter

Instructions:

Melt the butter in a large pot over medium high heat. Add in the onion, garlic, salt, pepper, nutmeg, and thyme. Sauté until the onions are soft and fragrant, about 3 minutes. Add in the tomatoes and stock, and bring to a boil. Reduce heat to low and simmer 20 minutes. Using an immersion blender, puree until smooth. Stir in the cream and simmer another 20 minutes. Serve warm.

> Nutrition: 135 calories, 10.1 g fat, 2.5 g protein, 6 g net carbs

Cream of Leek Soup

This soup is a French classic, and very comforting! Serve alongside a piece of crusty Low Carb Baguette for a classic French experience!

Servings: 6

Serving Size: about 1 ½ cups

Prep Time: 10 minutes

Cook Time: 40 minutes

Ingredients:

  1 leek, whites only, chopped

  ½ onion, diced

  1 clove garlic, minced

  4 cups chicken stock

  1 Tablespoon thyme

  1 cup cream

  ¼ cup butter

  1 teaspoon salt

  1 teaspoon pepper

  ½ cup gruyere, shredded

Instructions:

Melt the butter in a large pot over medium high heat. Add in the leek, onion, garlic, salt, pepper, and thyme. Sauté until the leeks and onions are soft and fragrant, about 5 minutes. Add in the stock, and bring to a boil. Reduce heat to low and simmer 20 minutes. Using an immersion blender, puree until smooth. Stir in the cream, and simmer another 20 minutes. Stir in the cheese. Serve warm.

  Nutrition: 175 calories, 14.5 g fat, 4.3 g protein, 3 g net carbs

Cream of Mushroom Soup

Mushrooms are incredibly low carb and high flavor, making them a great ingredient to incorporate into your keto meals! This soup is full of rich cream, parmesan cheese, and coconut oil for a great hit of fat.

Servings: 2

Serving Size: about 1 ½ cups

Prep Time: 10 minutes

Cook Time: 0 minutes

Ingredients:

  8 oz cremini mushrooms, sliced thinly

  1 stalk celery, chopped

  ½ onion, chopped

  1 Tablespoon coconut oil

  1 Tablespoon thyme, chopped

  1 teaspoon dried thyme

  ½ Tablespoon salt

½ Tablespoon pepper

½ cup vegetable stock or chicken stock

1 cup cream

3 Tablespoons parmesan cheese, grated

Instructions:

Preheat a medium sized pot over medium heat. Add in the coconut oil, mushrooms, celery, onion, thyme, salt and pepper. Sauté 2 minutes, until soft and fragrant. Add in the stock, and bring to a boil. Reduce heat to low, and simmer 30 minutes. Stir in the cream, and continue cooking another 10 minutes. Stir in the parmesan cheese. Taste, and season with salt and pepper. Serve hot, or transfer to an airtight container and store in the fridge for up to 3 weeks.

Nutrition: 222 calories, 15.6 g fat, 7.8 g protein, 11 g net carbs

Creamy Cauliflower and Seafood Chowder

This chowder is rich, creamy, and perfectly flavorful! This is a great way to use up leftover fish recipes like Red Pepper Cod!

Serving: 6

Serving Size: about ¾ cup

Prep Time: 5 minutes

Cook Time: 30 Minutes

Ingredients

4 slices bacon, diced

½ onion, diced

2 Tablespoons butter

1 Tablespoon olive oil

3 cloves garlic, minced

1 teaspoon paprika

1 teaspoon thyme

2 cups chicken stock

½ head cauliflower, chopped

1 cup heavy cream

¼ lb cooked white fish

3 scallops, cooked and diced

¼ lb shrimp, diced

¼ lb cooked crab meat, shredded

1 tomato, diced

Instructions

Preheat a large pot over medium heat. Drizzle in the olive oil, and melt in the butter. Cook the bacon bits for about a minute in the butter. Add the onion and garlic, along with the paprika and time, and sauté for a minute longer, until soft. Add in the cauliflower and stock, and bring to a boil. Reduce heat to low, and simmer 20 minutes. Using an immersion blender, puree until smooth. Add in the fish, tomato, and cream. Simmer another 5-10 minutes. Serve warm.

Nutrition: 540 calories, 52 g fat, 28 g protein, 7 g net carbs

Nicoise Salad

This salad seems complicated, but all of the individual components can be prepared in advance. The tuna can be cooked up to a day in advance and sliced right before serving, as can the hard boiled eggs. The dressing can be made up to a week in advance, as well. Cook the green beans in advance and keep them in an airtight container - you may want to do this in batches. Green beans make an excellent low carb count snacking option, and a wonderful addition to most salads!

Serving: 1

Serving Size: whole recipe

Prep Time: 5 minutes

Cook Time: 20 Minutes

Ingredients

1 8 oz ahi tuna steak

6 green beans

4 cherry tomatoes

2 eggs

¼ cucumber, sliced

1 cup kale, chopped

2 Tablespoons Dijon mustard

¼ cup olive oil

1 teaspoon dried thyme

Instructions

Bring a pot of water to a boil. Boil the eggs for about 6 minutes, to hard boil. Allow to cool fully before peeling. Pat the tuna dry, and season with salt and pepper. Preheat a small pan over medium high heat. Drizzle a bit of olive oil, and sear the ahi for about 1 minute per side. Transfer the seared ahi to a cutting board, and allow to cool fully before slicing. Bring another pot of salted water to a boil, and blanch the beans for about a minute. Drain, and transfer to an ice bath until ready to use. Next, whisk together the mustard, thyme and olive oil in a large bowl. Taste, and season with salt and pepper as needed. Toss the kale in the dressing, then transfer to a plate. Slice the ahi, and lay on top of the greens. Lay the beans, cucumber and tomato on top. Peel the eggs, slice them in half, and lay them on top of the salad. Serve immediately.

Nutrition: 273 calories, 20g fat, 23g protein, 2g net carbs

Italian Chopped Salad

This chopped salad is so easy to throw together, and super versatile! Add in your favorite marinated meats and veg to make this your own! This salad will keep in the fridge for up to 5 days, so make a big batch and have it on hand for snacking or fast lunch options.

Serving: 2

Serving Size: half recipe

Prep Time: 15 minutes

Cook Time: 0 minutes

Ingredients

12 Romaine leaves, chopped

2 oz prosciutto, sliced into ribbons

2 oz salami, chopped

¼ cup artichoke hearts, chopped

¼ cup olives

1 jalapeno, sliced

1 Tablespoon olive oil

1 Tablespoon lemon juice or white wine vinegar

1 Tablespoon Italian herbs

Instructions

In a large bowl, whisk together the olive oil, lemon juice and herbs. Toss in the rest of the ingredients, making sure everything is well mixed. Season with salt and pepper. Serve immediately, or store in an airtight container in the fridge for up to 5 days.

Nutrition: 469 calories, 44g fat, 14g protein, 4g net carbs

Cilantro Lime Shrimp and Avocado Salad

This salad is summer in a bowl! The creamy avocado stands up nicely to the tangy shrimp.

Serving: 1

Serving Size: whole recipe

Prep Time: 5 minutes

Cook Time: 5 Minutes

Ingredients

> 6 shrimp, deveined and peeled
>
> ½ lime, juice and zest
>
> 1 Tablespoon avocado oil
>
> ½ teaspoon garlic powder
>
> 2 Tablespoons cilantro, finely chopped
>
> ½ avocado, diced
>
> 1 teaspoon salt
>
> 1 jalapeno, diced
>
> 3 green onions, finely sliced
>
> 3 cherry tomatoes, cut in half

Instructions

Preheat a medium sized pan over medium high heat. Whisk together the lime juice, zest, avocado oil, garlic powder, and cilantro. Toss the shrimp in the marinade, and transfer to the pan. Cook about 1 minute per side, until the shrimp are opaque and firm. Mix the green onions, avocado, jalapeno and tomatoes together, and season with salt. Top with the shrimp. Serve immediately.

> Nutrition: 529 calories, 35.6 g fat, 26g protein, 5g net carbs

Scallop and Mushroom Salad with Goat Cheese Vinaigrette

This combo may seem a bit weird, but it works! The creamy scallops juxtapose nicely with the salty, fatty bacon and meaty mushrooms, and the creamy, tangy goat cheese vinaigrette brings it all together.

Serving: 2

Serving Size: half recipe

Prep Time: 5 minutes

Cook Time: 15 Minutes

Ingredients

> 6 scallops
>
> 2 slices bacon, diced
>
> 1 Tablespoon butter
>
> 1 cup mixed mushrooms, sliced
>
> 1 Tablespoon thyme
>
> 2 oz goat cheese

2 Tablespoons olive oil

1 cup arugula

½ lemon, juiced

Instructions

Preheat a medium pan over medium high heat. Cook the bacon bits with the butter, then remove from the pan and set aside. In the same pan, sauté the mushrooms with the thyme and a pinch of salt until soft and fragrant, about 3 minutes. Remove from the pan and set aside. Next, pat the scallops dry and season with salt and pepper. In the same pan, sear the scallops for about 2-3 minutes per side. Remove from the pan and set aside. Turn off the heat, and whisk the goat cheese, olive oil and lemon juice into the flavored butter. Spoon the goat cheese vinaigrette into a large bowl, and toss in the arugula, mushrooms and bacon. Toss well to combine. To serve, lay the dressed arugula onto two plates, and top with 3 scallops each. Serve warm.

Nutrition: 498 calories, 38.8 g fat, 32.7 g protein, 4.4 g net carbs

Egg Salad

This salad is an instant energy booster and a great grab and go lunch! Leftovers will stay good in the fridge for up to five days. Serve on lettuce wraps or with some fresh greens. Would taste good with crackers or Nordic seed bread, too.

Servings: 4

Serving Size: about ¼ cup

Prep Time: 10 minutes

Cook Time: 10 minutes

Ingredients:

8 eggs

½ cup mayonnaise

1 green onion, thinly sliced

1 teaspoon salt

Mustard

Dill pickles

Paprika for garnish

Instructions:

Put the eggs into a medium sized pot filled with water. Bring to a boil, and boil about 10 minutes, until the eggs are hard boiled (can be done up to three days in advance). Allow to cool, peel, and mash lightly in a bowl with the rest of the ingredients. Sprinkle with red paprika for a garnish. Serve immediately, or refrigerate up to 4 days.

Nutrition: 242 calories, 18.6g fat, 11.4 g protein, 8g net carbs

Chicken Salad

Classic chicken salad is a summertime staple. This recipe has celery and pecans for crunch. You can serve it alongside Nordic seed bread or Keto crackers. Roast or bake your chicken the night before, so it's ready for shredding in the morning.

Servings: 4

Serving Size: 1/2 cup

Prep Time: 10 minutes

Cook Time: 0 minutes

Ingredients:

> 3 cups cold shredded chicken
>
> 1/2 cup full fat mayonnaise
>
> 1 teaspoon Dijon mustard
>
> Juice from half a lemon
>
> 2 stalks celery, sliced
>
> ¼ cup chopped pecans
>
> 1.5 Tablespoons fresh chopped parsley
>
> 1 Tablespoon chopped dill
>
> Salt and pepper to taste

Instructions:

Combine all ingredients in a large bowl except for the chicken and the pecans. Stir thoroughly. Then add the chicken and toss. Finally, add the pecans and toss again. Taste for seasonings and adjust salt and pepper. Serve cold on lettuce or with crackers.

> Nutrition: 367 calories, 25g fat, 34g protein, 2g net carbs

Kale Salad

This low carb salad is just the thing to ensure you're getting the vitamins and minerals you need, while still watching your Macros! It's super crunchy, so it will keep in the fridge with the dressing for about a day without going soggy. This salad is great on its own, and goes well with chicken, pork, or steak.

Servings: 1

Serving Size: about 1 ½ cups

Prep Time: 10 minutes

Cook Time: 0 minutes

Ingredients:

1 cup kale, chopped

¼ red onion, sliced thinly

2 radishes, grated

2 Tablespoons olive oil

½ Tablespoon Dijon mustard

½ Tablespoon mayonnaise

1 teaspoon thyme

1 teaspoon salt

½ teaspoon Stevia

Instructions:

In a large bowl, whisk together the olive oil, Dijon, mayonnaise, thyme, salt and Stevia to make a dressing. Toss in the rest of the ingredients, and mix well. Serve immediately, or keep in an airtight container in the fridge for up to two days.

Nutrition: 322 calories, 30.9 g fat, 2.9 g protein, 9 g net carbs

Warm Zucchini and Goat Cheese Salad

This fabulous salad is low protein, high fat and amazingly flavorful!

Servings: 1

Serving Size: whole recipe

Prep Time: 10 minutes

Cook Time: 30 minutes

Ingredients:

½ zucchini, sliced

1 Tablespoon olive oil, divided

1/2 cup basil, chopped

1 handful parsley, chopped

1 teaspoon Italian herbs (basil, oregano, parsley)

1 clove garlic, minced

½ Tablespoon white wine vinegar

¼ cup sun dried tomatoes

2 oz goat cheese

¼ cup walnuts

Instructions:

Preheat the oven to 375F. Toss the zucchini in one Tablespoon of olive oil and season with salt, pepper, and the Italian herbs. Bake in the oven for 10 minutes. Meanwhile, whisk together the garlic, herbs, white wine vinegar, and second Tablespoon of olive oil. Toss the rest of the ingredients in, and mix well. Serve immediately.

Nutrition: 395 calories, 35.5 g fat, 14.8 g protein, 6 g net carbs

Green Goddess Dressing

This dressing is high fat and high flavor! Perfect for topping on any salad, or using as a dip for veggies!

Servings: 4

Serving Size: ¼ cup

Prep Time: 10 minutes

Cook Time: 0 minutes

Ingredients:

2 avocados

¼ cup olive oil

1 Tablespoon thyme

1 Tablespoon white wine vinegar

1 teaspoon salt

Instructions:

In a blender or food processor, combine all ingredients until smooth. Store in an airtight container in the fridge for up to a week.

Nutrition: 316 calories, 32 g fat, 2 g protein, 2 g net carbs

Thai Coconut Dressing

This dressing is full of coconut milk and exotic flavor! Perfect for dressing on top of Asian style salads, and also works great as a marinade for chicken or pork!

Servings: 4

Serving Size: ¼ cup

Prep Time: 10 minutes

Cook Time: 0 minutes

Ingredients:

1 avocado

2 cans coconut milk

3 red chilis, minced

1 clove garlic, minced

Handful cilantro, chopped

1 teaspoon ginger, minced

3 green onions, chopped

Instructions:

In a blender or food processor, combine all ingredients until smooth. Store in an airtight container in the fridge for up to a week.

Nutrition: 247 calories, 25 g fat, 2.6 g protein, 3.8 g net carbs

Asian Nut Dressing

This dressing is spicy, creamy, and super flavorful! It works well on Asian style salads as well as a marinade for beef, chicken or pork.

Servings: 4

Serving Size: ¼ cup

Prep Time: 10 minutes

Cook Time: 0 minutes

Ingredients:

½ cup almond butter

½ cup coconut milk

2 limes, juice and zest

Handful cilantro, chopped

3 green onions, chopped

4 red chilis, minced

¼ cup sesame oil

Instructions:

In a blender or food processor, combine all ingredients until smooth. Store in an airtight container in the fridge for up to a week.

Nutrition: 205 calories, 21.9 g fat, 1.3 g protein, 1 g net carbs

Cilantro Lime Dressing

This zingy dressing is perfect for Steak and Avocado Salad, but will work on any Southwest inspired salad creations!

Servings: 4

Serving Size: ¼ cup

Prep Time: 10 minutes

Cook Time: 0 minutes

Ingredients:

> ½ cup avocado oil
>
> 4 limes, juice and zest
>
> 2 cups fresh cilantro, chopped
>
> 1 jalapeno, chopped

Instructions:

In a blender or food processor, combine all ingredients until smooth. Store in an airtight container in the fridge for up to a week.

> Nutrition: 60 calories, 3.9 g fat, 1g protein, 4 g net carbs

Lemon Thyme Vinaigrette

This dressing is classically French and really yummy! Use it to on a simple green salad, or as a marinade for fish!

Servings: 4

Serving Size: ¼ cup

Prep Time: 10 minutes

Cook Time: 0 minutes

Ingredients:

> ½ cup olive oil
>
> 4 lemons, juice and zest
>
> 4 large stems thyme, chopped
>
> 1 Tablespoon Dijon mustard

Instructions:

In a blender or food processor, combine all ingredients until smooth. Store in an airtight container in the fridge for up to a week.

> Nutrition: 60 calories, 3.9 g fat, 1g protein, 2 g net carbs

Pork Chopped Salad

Using leftover pork chops, you can create this fun, easy salad very quickly! Switch up the ingredients to really make this meat-filled salad your own!

Serving: 1

Serving Size: whole recipe

Prep Time: 15 minutes

Cook Time: 0 minutes

Ingredients

> 2 cooked pork chops, 1" thick (4 oz each)
>
> 1/4 cup kale, chopped
>
> 3 cherry tomatoes, halved
>
> 1 egg, hardboiled
>
> ½ cucumber, sliced
>
> 2 Tablespoons olive oil
>
> 1 Tablespoon white wine vinegar
>
> 2 teaspoons Dijon mustard
>
> 1 teaspoon thyme
>
> 1 teaspoon salt
>
> 1 teaspoon pepper

Instructions

Start by slicing the pork chop thinly, and setting aside. Next, whisk together the olive oil, vinegar, mustard, thyme, salt and pepper in a large bowl, and add in the kale. Toss well to combine. Mix in the cherry tomatoes, cucumber and pork slices. Slice the peeled hard boiled egg in half, and toss it into the salad. Serve immediately, or keep in the fridge for up to 24 hours.

> Nutrition: 681 calories, 57.9 g fat, 29 g protein, 9 g net carbs

Avocado and Chicken Salad

This rich, creamy salad can be eaten on its own, or wrapped in lettuce for a healthy, hand-held option! Switch up the seasoning to suit your own tastes - if you like things on the spicier side, add jalapeno or hot sauce! If you like an herbier salad, add in your favorite fresh or dried herbs!

Serving: 1

Serving Size: whole recipe

Prep Time: 5 minutes

Cook Time: 0 minutes

Ingredients

> 1 avocado, diced
>
> 4 oz chicken breast, cooked and sliced
>
> 1 Tablespoon coconut oil

2 teaspoons salt

1 Tablespoon lime juice

1 teaspoon lime zest

Instructions

Mix together all ingredient in a bowl, making sure to mash the avocado and chicken together to make a creamy bind. Taste, and adjust seasoning as needed. Serve immediately, or enjoy within 4 hours.

Nutrition: 663 calories, 55 g fat, 28 protein, 6 g net carbs

Asian Salad

This super simple salad is made with Asian Nut Dressing and super fresh ingredients. If you wish, you can add a piece of chicken or pork on top!

Servings: 2

Serving Size: ½ recipe

Prep Time: 10 minutes

Cook Time: 10 minutes

Ingredients:

2 servings Asian Nut Dressing

¼ cup bean sprouts

¼ carrot, grated

¼ red pepper, sliced thinly

1 avocado, diced

3 green onions, thinly sliced

1 cup shiitake mushrooms

2 Tablespoons sesame oil

Instructions:

Preheat oven to 375F. Toss the mushrooms in the sesame oil, and lay out on a baking sheet. Roast for 10 minutes. Meanwhile, toss together the rest of the ingredients. Make sure the dressing has fully coated each piece. When the mushrooms are done, toss them in right away. Serve immediately, or keep in an airtight container for up to 3 days.

Nutrition: 579 calories, 55.4 g fat, 5 g protein, 9 g net carbs

Lemon Thyme Salmon Salad

This salad is so lovely and delicate, and the perfect lunch for a warm summer day!

Serving: 2

Serving Size: 1 fillet fish

Prep Time: 5 minutes

Cook Time: 25 minutes

Ingredients

> 2 4 oz pieces salmon
>
> 1 Tablespoon olive oil
>
> 1 teaspoon thyme
>
> 1 teaspoon nutmeg
>
> ½ head cauliflower, cut into florets
>
> 4 green beans
>
> ½ tomato, cut into wedges
>
> 1 egg, hardboiled and cut in half
>
> ½ green pepper, sliced into strips
>
> 2 cups arugula
>
> 2 servings Lemon Thyme Vinaigrette

Instructions

Preheat oven to 350F. Brush the oil over the fish, and season with the thyme, nutmeg and a pinch of salt. Bake 25 minutes. Meanwhile, bring a large pot of salted water to a boil, and cook the cauliflower florets for 3 minutes, to blanche. Transfer to an ice bath. Cook the green beans in the same water for 1 minute, and then transfer to an ice bath. Toss the arugula with the dressing, and lay onto two plates. Place one half of the hardboiled egg onto each plate, followed by a few tomato wedges, the green beans and cauliflower. Top with the fish. Serve immediately.

> Nutrition: 402 calories, 21.1 g fat, 41.7 g protein, 9.1 g net carbs

Baja Style Halibut Salad

This salad is bright and fresh and full of color! Leftover fish can be used in lettuce wraps to make Fish Tacos.

Serving: 2

Serving Size: 1 fillet fish

Prep Time: 5 minutes

Cook Time: 25 minutes

Ingredients

> 2 4 oz pieces of halibut
>
> 1 Tablespoon olive oil

1 teaspoon oregano

1 teaspoon garlic powder

1 teaspoon salt

2 cups arugula

1 tomato, diced

½ bell pepper, diced

1 jalapeno, diced

¼ red onion, sliced

1 avocado, diced

2 servings Cilantro Lime Dressing

Instructions

Preheat oven to 350F. Brush the oil over the fish, and season with the oregano, garlic, and a pinch of salt. Bake 25 minutes. Toss the arugula with the dressing, and lay onto two plates. Top with the remaining veg. Top with the fish. Serve immediately or keep leftovers in an airtight container in the fridge for up to two days.

Nutrition: 740 calories, 40 g fat, 95 g protein, 7 g net carbs

Steak and Avocado Salad

This salad is light and flavorful and full of good fat! Perfect for a cold summer lunch!

Servings: 2

Serving Size: Half recipe

Prep Time: 10 minutes

Cook Time: 15 minutes

Ingredients:

1/4 lb flank steak, cut into strips

1 Tablespoon olive oil

1 Tablespoon jalapeno powder

1 teaspoon salt

¼ red onion, sliced

1 avocado, diced

½ tomato, diced

1 serving Cilantro Lime Dressing

Instructions:

Preheat a large pan over medium heat. Toss the steak in the olive oil and jalapeno powder, and fry until fully cooked- about 3 minutes. Transfer to a bowl with the rest of the ingredients, and toss well to combine. Serve immediately. Could also be wrapped in lettuce leaves with Monterey Jack cheese and salsa to create lettuce wraps.

Nutrition: 663 calories, 44 g fat, 50 g protein, 7 g net carbs

Pork and Poultry

Jerk Chicken

Jerk Chicken is deliciously flavorful and full of good fat! Enjoy over cauliflower rice for a Keto friendly Caribbean experience!

Serving: 4

Serving Size: 1 chicken thigh

Prep Time: 5 minutes

Cook Time: 45 minutes

Ingredients

- 4 chicken thighs, bone in skin on

- 3 Tablespoons allspice

- ½ Tablespoon ginger

- 2 cloves garlic, minced

- ½ onion, diced

- 2 scotch bonnets, minced

- 1 teaspoon cinnamon

- 1 Tablespoon thyme

- ¼ cup dry white wine

- 2 cups chicken stock

- 2 Tablespoons coconut oil

Instructions

Preheat the oven to 375F. Combine the allspice, ginger, cinnamon and thyme together, and rub into the chicken. Preheat a Dutch oven on the stove over medium high heat, and melt in the coconut oil. Add the onion, garlic, and scotch bonnets, and sauté 1 minute. Add in the chicken and stock, and cover. Transfer to the oven, and cook 40 minutes.

Nutrition: 524 calories, 33.9 g fat, 44 g protein, 5 g net carbs

Thai Chicken Coconut Red Curry

This is such a fragrant and easy dish, where you can make substitutions depending on what you have. You can use shrimp, beef, or pork instead of the chicken. Try yellow or green curry paste instead of the red. Use any combination of fresh Keto vegetables you prefer.

Serving: 4

Serving Size: ¼ recipe

Prep Time: 10 minutes

Cook Time: 20 minutes

Ingredients

> 1 Tablespoon olive oil
>
> 2 Tablespoons red curry paste (or yellow or green)
>
> 13.5 ounce can of full fat coconut milk
>
> ½ cup chicken broth
>
> 1/8 teaspoon Stevia
>
> 1 Tablespoon fish sauce
>
> 1 1b boneless skinless chicken cut into 1" pieces
>
> 3 cups assorted bite-size cut fresh vegetables (green peppers, broccoli,
>
> > cauliflower, onion, bok choy, tomatoes, zucchini, etc.)
>
> 1 Tablespoon thinly sliced fresh basil (optional)
>
> Squeeze of fresh lime

Instructions

Put your large skillet or wok on medium heat. Heat the olive oil. When warm, add the curry paste and stir fry with a wooden spoon for 1 ½ - 2 minutes until fragrant. Pour in entire can of coconut milk and the chicken broth. Raise the temperature to medium-high. Bring to a simmer. Then stir in the Stevia (no more than 1/8 teaspoon or to taste) and the fish sauce until well blended. Add the meat and all of the vegetables and stir to coat everything in the curry. Simmer uncovered for 5-7 minutes until the chicken is cooked through. Remove from heat. Stir in the basil and a squeeze of fresh lime. Could also add sliced spring onion and a sprinkle of fresh finely chopped cilantro.

> Nutrition: 310 calories, 26 g fat, 14 g protein, 7 g net carbs

Indian Butter Chicken with Roasted Cauliflower

If you live in a cold climate, there is nothing more warming or comforting than Indian food! You can find the garam masala at Asian stores or online. This recipe is packed with chicken, butter, and spices. It's delicious. Use ghee to increase your fat intake.

Servings: 6

Serving Size: 1/6 recipe

Prep Time: 30 minutes

Cook Time: 30 minutes

Ingredients

  1 2/3 lbs boneless chicken thighs

  1 tomato, cored

  1 yellow onion

  2 Tablespoons ginger

  2 garlic cloves, peeled

  1 Tablespoon tomato paste

  1 Tablespoon garam masala seasoning

  ½ Tablespoon ground coriander (cilantro)

  ½ Tablespoon chili powder

  1 teaspoon salt

  ¾ cup heavy cream

  3 oz butter or Indian ghee

For Cauliflower:

  1 lb cauliflower, chopped into bite size pieces

  ½ teaspoon turmeric

  ½ tablespoon coriander seed

  ½ teaspoon salt

  ¼ teaspoon black pepper

  2 oz melted butter

Instructions

In a blender or food processor, blend the tomato, onion, ginger, garlic, tomato paste, and the spices – garam masala, coriander, chili powder, and salt. Blend until smooth. Add the heavy cream and stir in. Pour into a bowl and add the cut up chicken until well coated. Cover with plastic wrap and marinate in the fridge for at least 20 minutes. You could marinate for several hours to infuse the flavor. When ready to cook, heat up a large frying pan over medium high heat with 1 ounce of the butter. Add the chicken to the pan and fry on each side for several minutes. Then pour the rest of the marinade over the chicken, together with the other 2 ounces of butter. Turn heat down to medium and let simmer for 15 minutes until chicken is fully cooked. For the cauliflower, preheat your oven to 400F. Spread the chopped cauliflower over a foil cookie sheet or baking tray.

Sprinkle the seasonings and butter over. Bake for 15 minutes. Serve the butter chicken over the cauliflower and garnish with fresh cilantro and plain unsweetened yogurt.

Nutrition: 592 calories, 52g fat, 24g protein, 6g net carbs

Chicken Avocado Pesto Pasta

This is a quick and easy dinner recipe that from start to finish is on the table in 30 minutes. It uses zucchini 'zoodles' to mimic pasta!

Serving: 2

Serving Size: half recipe

Prep Time: 15 minutes

Cook Time: 15 minutes

Ingredients

2 zucchinis, spiralized or cut into ribbons

8 oz chicken breast, sliced

1 Tablespoon oregano

1 Tablespoon garlic powder

1 Tablespoon coconut oil

1 avocado

2 Tablespoons extra virgin olive oil

1/2 cup water

1/2 cup basil

salt and pepper to taste

Instructions

In a blender or food processor, blend together the avocado, olive oil, water, and basil. Set aside. In a medium pan over medium high heat, melt the coconut oil. Add in the chicken slices, oregano and garlic powder, tossing frequently and cooking until done, about 8 minutes. Add in the avocado mixture and zucchini noodles, tossing well to combine. Cook until heated through, about 7 minutes.

Nutrition: 440 calories, 40g fat, 36g protein, 3g net carbs

Chicken Kababs

Kababs are delicious, and make a great summer treat when grilled on the BBQ! Serve them on their own with a dipping sauce (such as Green Tahini) or on top of greens for a complete meal!

Serving: 4

Serving Size: 1 skewer

Prep Time: 10 minutes

Cook Time: 30 minutes

Ingredients

>4 3 oz boneless skinless chicken thighs, chopped into chunks

>¼ red onion, sliced into chunks

>½ bell pepper, sliced into chunks

>1 Tablespoon salt

>1 Tablespoon pepper

>1 Tablespoon paprika

>1 teaspoon cumin

>3 Tablespoons olive oil

Instructions

Preheat the oven to 350F. Toss all ingredients together in a bowl, making sure the oil coats everything well. Using four skewers, skewer the meat and veggies evenly onto each skewer. Bake for 30 minutes, until the meat is cooked through and the veggies are soft.

>Nutrition: 270 calories, 17.2 g fat, 25 g protein, 2 g net carbs

Chicken Kale Wrap

This is a super simple recipe to throw together using leftover cooked chicken and a few simple ingredients! It makes a great lunch, or a quick weeknight dinner.

Serving: 1

Serving Size: 1 wrap

Prep Time: 5 minutes

Cook Time: 30 minutes

Ingredients

>2 large kale leaves

>4 oz chicken breast, cooked and sliced

>¼ red pepper, sliced

>2 Tablespoons tahini

Instructions

Start by washing and drying the kale leaves, and laying them out on a piece of parchment, so they overlap in the middle. Lay the chicken and pepper slices over top, and drizzle liberally with tahini. Season with salt and pepper, and roll the kale to make a wrap. Serve immediately, or keep wrapped in the parchment in the fridge for up to 24 hours.

Nutrition: 415 calories, 32.1g fat, 26.3 g protein, 5.3 g net carbs

Goat Cheese Stuffed Chicken Breasts

These chicken breasts are elegant and delicious! They can be served hot or cold, and make a great addition to salads.

Serving: 2

Serving Size: 1 chicken breast

Prep Time: 15 minutes

Cook Time: 30 minutes

Ingredients

> 2 6 oz chicken breasts
>
> 6 oz goat cheese
>
> 1 Tablespoon cream
>
> 1 Tablespoon dried thyme
>
> 1 Tablespoon smoked paprika
>
> 1 Tablespoon butter

Instructions

Preheat the oven to 350F. Slice the chicken breast open like a book, and place it between two pieces of plastic wrap. Pound lightly to flatten slightly, and transfer the flattened breast to a baking sheet lined with parchment. Continue on with the second breast. Next, beat together the goat cheese, cream, thyme and paprika with a bit of black pepper. Spoon the mixture evenly into the center of each breast, and roll them up. Next, beat together the butter with a bit more pepper, paprika and thyme, and spread the mixture all over the outside of the chicken to coat. Bake the chicken in the center of the oven for 30 minutes. Allow to rest 10 minutes, then slice into medallions.

Nutrition: 646 calories, 44.5 g fat, 55.9 g protein, 3 g net carbs

Beef and Lamb

Beef Stuffed Tomatoes

This Middle Eastern classic is a fun dinner or lunch option! Serve it with a side of greens or on top of cauliflower rice.

Serving: 2

Serving Size: 1 tomato

Prep Time: 5 minutes

Cook Time: 25 minutes

Ingredients

> ½ lb ground beef
>
> 1 Tablespoon olive oil
>
> 1 teaspoon thyme
>
> 1 teaspoon paprika
>
> 1 clove garlic, minced
>
> ½ onion, diced
>
> 2 large red tomatoes

Instructions

Hollow out the centers of the tomatoes by removing the core and the soft insides. Preheat the oven to 375F. Preheat a pan over medium high heat, and drizzle in the olive oil. Add in the onion with a pinch of salt and the spices, and sauté for about a minute. Add in the beef, and cook until done, about 3-4 minutes. Spoon the mixture into the hollowed out tomatoes, and place them onto a baking sheet lined with parchment. Bake 18-20 minutes, until the tomatoes have softened and blistered slightly. Serve warm. Keep leftovers in an airtight container for up to four days.

> Nutrition: 350 calories, 15.5g fat, 36g protein, 5 g net carbs

Greek Lamb Burger

This lamb burger combines classic Greek flavors, giving you a fun international twist on a basic burger! This is a bun less burger, so make sure you've got your knife and fork (and appetite!) ready!

Serving: 2

Serving Size: 2 Patties

Prep Time: 5 minutes

Cook Time: 15 minutes

Ingredients

> 1 lb ground lamb
>
> 1 cup shredded romaine lettuce
>
> 2 teaspoons salt
>
> 1 teaspoon white pepper
>
> 1 Tablespoon coconut oil
>
> 1 cup Greek yogurt
>
> 1/4 English cucumber, diced

1 Tablespoon of fresh dill

1 clove garlic, minced

1 teaspoon salt

Instructions

In a large bowl combine the ground lamb, paprika, sea salt and pepper and form 4 patties. Heat a pan on medium heat and add the coconut oil. Once the coconut oil has melted place the burger patties in the pan and cook for about 5 minutes per side. Meanwhile peel and shred the cucumber and then combine it with all of the other ingredients to make the Tzatziki sauce. To serve, top one patty with the tzatziki and lettuce, and top with the second patty. Serve immediately.

Nutrition: 542 calories, 40g fat, 36g protein, 5g net carbs

Lamb Chops with Buttery Mustard Sauce

Lamb and mustard are a match made in heaven! Serve alongside asparagus or a fresh salad with light dressing.

Serving: 2

Serving Size: 1 chop

Prep Time: 5 minutes

Cook Time: 25 minutes

Ingredients

2 6 oz lamb chops

4 Tablespoons butter

1 stem thyme

3 Tablespoons Dijon mustard

1 Tablespoon salt

1 Tablespoon pepper

Instructions

Preheat oven to 350F. Season the lamb chops with salt and pepper, and lay on a baking sheet lined with parchment. Bake for 20 minutes, until cooked through. Melt the butter in a saucepan over medium high heat. Add the mustard and thyme. Cook for 30 minutes, stirring occasionally. Remove the thyme stem, and spoon the sauce over the lamb chops.

Nutrition: 429 calories, 27g fat, 25g protein, 9g net carbs

Walnut and Pork Stuffed Lamb Tenderloin

Lamb tenderloin is a sophisticated showpiece dish that is perfect for entertaining! The walnut stuffing is savory, fatty, and complements the lamb perfectly. Serve this masterpiece of a dish with a side of Butter Tossed Asparagus for a beautiful keto-friendly masterpiece! Leftovers keep really well as well, and make a great addition to sandwiches and salads.

Servings: 6

Serving Size: 1 piece

Prep Time: 10 minutes

Cook Time: 45 minutes

Ingredients:

> 12 oz lamb tenderloin
>
> 1 cup walnuts, chopped
>
> 2 oz ground pork
>
> 1 Tablespoon thyme
>
> 1 Tablespoon butter
>
> 1 Tablespoon salt
>
> 1 Tablespoon pepper
>
> 1 teaspoon nutmeg

Instructions:

Preheat oven to 350F. In a pan over medium high heat, melt the butter and add the pork, thyme, nutmeg, salt and pepper. Cook 2-3 minutes, until the pork is cooked. Add in the walnuts, and cook another 2-3 minutes. Let cool fully. Next, make an incision down the length of the tenderloin, and roll your knife through the middle of the tenderloin to open it up. Fill the center of the lamb with the walnut and pork mixture, and seal it back up. Using some butcher twine, tie the tenderloin to keep the stuffing in place. Season the lamb with salt and pepper, and lay it on a baking sheet lined with parchment. Bake in the oven for 35-40 minutes. Let rest for 15 minutes. Slice into medallions and serve.

> Nutrition: 800 calories, 66.6 g fat, 45.5 g protein, 0.2 g net carbs

Beef Kababs

Kababs are delicious, and make a great summer treat when grilled on the BBQ! Serve them on their own with a dipping sauce (such as Green Tahini) or on top of greens for a complete meal.

Serving: 4

Serving Size: 1 skewer

Prep Time: 10 minutes

Cook Time: 30 minutes

Ingredients

> ½ lb flank steak, chopped into chunks
>
> ¼ red onion, sliced into chunks
>
> ½ bell pepper, sliced into chunks

1 Tablespoon salt

1 Tablespoon pepper

1 Tablespoon paprika

1 teaspoon cumin

3 Tablespoons olive oil

Instructions

Preheat the oven to 350F. Toss all ingredients together in a bowl, making sure the oil coats everything well. Using four skewers, skewer the meat and veg evenly onto each skewer. Bake for 30 minutes, until the meat is cooked through and the veg are soft.

Nutrition: 219 calories, 15.7 g fat, 16g protein, 2 g net carbs

Basic Burger Patties

The burger patty recipe that works for any burger! Make a bunch of these, and keep them wrapped individually in the freezer! They can be thawed and baked in a 375F oven for 15 minutes, making it quick and fast to have a great burger anytime!

Serving: 12

Serving Size: 1 patty

Prep Time: 15 minutes

Cook Time: 30 minutes

Ingredients

6 lbs ground beef

2 Tablespoons salt

1 Tablespoon garlic powder

2 teaspoons cayenne

3 eggs

Instructions

Preheat oven to 350F. In a large bowl, combine all ingredients well. For 12 equal size patties, and press them onto a baking sheet lined with parchment. Bake for 25-30 minutes, until fully cooked. Serve immediately with your preferred toppings, or allow to cool and wrap individually in plastic wrap to freeze. If frozen, enjoy within 2 months.

Nutrition: 437 calories, 15.2g fat, 70 g protein, 0.2 g net carbs

Keto Chinese Beef and Broccoli

This quick dish couldn't be easier or more flavorful. It's packed with delicious, light Asian flavors, crunchy broccoli, and hearty beef. In 30 minutes or less, you'll have a quick dinner on the table that kids will like, too.

Serving: 4

Serving Size: ¼ of bowl

Prep Time: 15 minutes

Cook Time: 10 minutes

Ingredients

>   1 lb beef (sirloin or skirt steak)

>   1 or 2 heads of broccoli, cut into small florets

>   2 cloves garlic, minced

>   1 Tablespoon ginger

For marinade:

>   1 Tablespoon soy sauce

>   1 Tablespoon sesame oil

>   ½ teaspoon salt

>   ¼ teaspoon black pepper

For sauce:

>   2 Tablespoons soy sauce

>   1 Tablespoon fish sauce

>   2 teaspoons sesame oil

>   ¼ teaspoon black pepper

Instructions

Slice the beef into ¼" thick pieces. Marinate in the marinade ingredients. Heat up a pot of water until boiling and briefly cook broccoli until crunchy and tender. Drain and set aside. Heat up a wok over medium heat using 1 ½ Tablespoons of ghee or olive oil. Add the marinated beef and spread the beef over the bottom of the pan and cook until the edges are crispy. Flip beef over and finish cooking. Add broccoli and cook another several minutes, then add the sauce ingredients. Toss everything to combine with sauce. Could garnish with toasted sesame seeds and sliced green onion.

>   Nutrition: 273 calories, 17 g fat, 24 g protein, 3 g net carbs

Beef Fajita Bowl

Hungry for Mexican food? Then you'll love making this yummy Beef Fajita Bowl. Leftovers can be made into wraps or a salad, so you actually get three meals in one, only cooking once! Perfect for summer.

Servings: 4

Serving Size: 1 portion

Prep Time: 15 minutes

Cook Time: 15 minutes

Ingredients

      1 lb steak, sliced into strips

      2 teaspoons olive oil

      2 green bell peppers, chopped

      1 onion, chopped

      1 clove garlic, minced

      1 teaspoon chili powder

      1 teaspoon ground cumin

      ½ teaspoon paprika

      ½ teaspoon salt

Instructions

Place your 12" skillet on medium heat and add 1 of the teaspoons of olive oil. When pan is warm, add steak and saute until half cooked, about 5-6 minutes. Then add second teaspoon of olive oil and the peppers, onion, and garlic. Saute several minutes, then add the chili powder and cumin and paprika. Cook until steak is completely cooked and the veggies are crisp tender, about another 4-5 minutes. Sprinkle with salt. Divide amongst four bowls and serve hot with salsa, sour cream, and fresh cilantro. As an option, you could add some chopped Thai red chilis for some more heat.

      Nutrition: 360 calories, 12 g fat, 48 g protein, 11 g net carbs

Beef Fajita Lettuce Wraps

Using leftovers from the Beef Fajita Bowl, these fun little wraps are the perfect way to satisfy any taco cravings! They make a very portable lunch, dinner or snack, and are a snap to make! You can leave the fajita filling cold for a refreshing, easy lunch, or heat it up and build your fajitas one by one- the choice is up to you!

Serving: 1

Serving Size: 4 wraps

Prep Time: 15 minutes

Cook Time: 2 minutes

Ingredients

      1 serving Beef Fajita Bowl

      4 large leaves iceberg or Romaine lettuce

      2 Tablespoons salsa, for dipping (optional)

      2 Tablespoons guacamole, for dipping

Instructions

If you prefer your fajita filling to be hot, microwave covered on high for 2 minutes. If not, move on to the next step. Spoon the filling into the lettuce leaf, folding the base slightly to keep everything inside. Spoon the salsa and guacamole on top, and dive in! Serve immediately.

> Nutrition: 513 calories, 37 g fat, 34 g protein, 9 g net carbs

Lettuce Wrapped Lamb Burgers

These lettuce wrapped burgers are a convenient way to bring your bun less burger to work or school for a quick, easy, portable lunch! Using leftover lamb burgers and tzatziki sauce, the crispy romaine lettuce holds it all together, while the addition of sliced bell peppers adds a bit of color and interest to the meal!

Serving: 1

Serving Size: 2 burgers

Prep Time: 15 minutes

Cook Time: 1 minute

Ingredients

> 1 serving Greek Lamb Burger
>
> 1 serving of Tzatziki (from same recipe)
>
> 4-6 large iceberg lettuce leaves
>
> ¼ red bell pepper, finely sliced

Instructions

Warm the burger patties by microwaving on high for 1 minute. Next, lay two or three pieces of lettuce out evenly, and spoon the tzatziki sauce over it. Top with the burger patty and pepper slices, and fold the lettuce leaves over to create a wrap. Do the same with the second burger, and remaining lettuce leaves, tzatziki and peppers. Serve immediately.

> Nutrition: 513 calories, 37 g fat, 34 g protein, 9 g net carbs

Steak and Avocado Taco Cups

Yummy grilled steak and diced avocado make a great Southwest style filling for these crispy taco cups! You'll never miss taco shells again, once you've had these!

Serving: 1

Serving Size: 4 tacos

Prep Time: 15 minutes

Cook Time: 5 minutes

Ingredients

> 1 hard boiled egg, chopped

¼ lb flank steak, sliced

1 diced avocado

1 Tablespoon lemon juice

2 teaspoons salt

1 Tablespoon olive oil

2 oz Monterey Jack Cheese, shredded

2 Tablespoons salsa

Instructions

Season the steak with salt and pepper. Over medium heat, preheat a skillet with the olive oil. Sear each side of the steak for about 3 – 5 minutes, cooking to medium rare. Take the steak out and let rest for at least 10 minutes before slicing. Toss the avocado with lemon juice in a bowl. Mix in the egg and toss in the steak. Season with more salt and pepper. Preheat the oven to 375F. Lay the cheese into 4 even piles on a baking sheet lined with parchment, and bake 5 minutes until the cheese has started to melt and bubble. Allow the cheese to cool slightly, and then carefully pick up each mound and place it into a muffin tin to cool for another 10-15 minutes, until cool and hardened. Spoon the salad into each cup. Top with salsa. Serve immediately.

Nutrition: 650 calories, 53 g fat, 40 g protein, 6 g net carbs

Cheese Stuffed Meatballs

Think of these like little meaty fat bombs! These meatballs are perfect when you just want a little something, but also work really well as an appetizer or main. Make a big batch and freeze them, for an easy meatball fix anytime!

Serving: 4

Serving Size: 3 meatballs

Prep Time: 10 minutes

Cook Time: 25 minutes

Ingredients

1 ½ lbs ground beef

4 oz cheddar cheese, shredded

4 Tablespoons parmesan cheese, shredded

½ teaspoon salt

½ teaspoon pepper

Instructions

Preheat the oven to 350F. Mix all ingredients together in a bowl. Roll out 12 equal sized balls. Lay the balls onto a baking sheet lined with parchment, and bake 25 minutes until the meatballs are browned and cooked through.

If freezing, allow to cool fully and store in an airtight container for up to three months. To reheat from frozen, allow to thaw in the fridge overnight and bake 20 minutes at 350F. Serve warm.

Nutrition: 440 calories, 28 g fat, 46 g protein,2 g net carbs

Cheese Stuffed Burgers

These burgers are rich, and full of gooey cheese! Serve in a lettuce wrap, or on their own topped with tomato, onion and pickles for a decadent burger experience!

Servings: 4

Serving Size: 1 patty

Prep Time: 10 minutes

Cook Time: 35 minutes

Ingredients:

> 1 lb ground beef
>
> 1 Tablespoon onion powder
>
> ½ Tablespoon garlic powder
>
> 1 teaspoon cayenne powder
>
> 1 Tablespoon salt
>
> 1 Tablespoon pepper
>
> 4 cups cheddar cheese, shredded

Instructions:

Preheat oven to 350F. Mix the beef and spices together, and form into four patties. Press ¼ cup cheese into the center of each patty, forming the meat around it. Bake in the oven for 20 minutes. Serve warm or keep in an airtight container in the fridge for 8 days.

Nutrition: 681 calories, 44.7 g fat, 63.1 g protein, 3.7 g net carbs

Beef Vindaloo

Beef Vindaloo is a spicy, tomato based Indian stew that is rich in flavor. Serve with Cauliflower Rice!

Servings: 2

Serving Size: 1 cup

Prep Time: 60 minutes

Cook Time: 25 minutes

Ingredients:

> ½ lb flank steak, cut into chunks
>
> 1 Tablespoon olive oil

¼ cup butter or ghee

2 stalks celery, chopped

¼ onion, chopped

3 cloves garlic, minced

1" piece ginger, minced

2 tomatoes, chopped

1 teaspoon red wine vinegar

2 teaspoons cayenne pepper

4 red chilies, minced (optional)

1 cup beef stock

1 cup heavy cream

Instructions:

Mix together the olive oil, garlic, ginger, vinegar, cayenne and chilies. Add in the beef, and mix well. Let sit for 20 minutes, or overnight. Heat a large pot over medium heat. Add in the butter or ghee, and sauté the tomatoes and onion until soft- about 5 minutes. Add in the beef and marinade, and toss well to combine. Cook 3 minutes. Add the beef stock, and bring to a boil. Reduce heat to low, and simmer 20 minutes. Stir in the cream, and cook 10 minutes longer. Serve warm or keep in an airtight container in the fridge for up to 7 days.

Nutrition: 436 calories, 30.4 g fat, 35 g protein, 3.5 g net carbs

Beef Stew

This stew is warm and hearty, and really yummy!

Servings: 4

Serving Size: 1 cup

Prep Time: 10 minutes

Cook Time: 55 minutes

Ingredients:

1 lb flank steak, cut into chunks

1 Tablespoon olive oil

1 Tablespoon thyme

1 Tablespoon salt

4 cups beef stock

2 Tablespoons butter

1 carrot, chopped

2 stalks celery, chopped

1 14.5 oz can diced tomatoes

¼ onion, chopped

2 cloves garlic, minced

2 Tablespoons Worcestershire sauce

½ cup red wine (optional)

1 cup heavy cream

Instructions:

Preheat a large pot over medium heat. Drizzle the oil, and brown the beef on all sides- about 4 minutes. Remove from pan and set aside. In the same pot, melt in the butter and sauté the vegetables with the salt, until soft - about 3 minutes. Add in the herbs. Return the beef back to the pot. Add the stock and Worcestershire sauce and wine. Bring to a boil, then reduce heat to low. Simmer 25 minutes. Stir in the cream, and simmer another 15 minutes. You could also make this in a crockpot! After browning the beef, add the rest of the ingredients (except cream) to the crockpot and cook on low 4-6 hours. Turn heat off, let sit for 30 minutes to cool down, then add the heavy cream.

Nutrition: 450 calories, 30.4 g fat, 35 g protein, 4.5 g net carbs

Seafood

Red Pepper Cod

This easy, classic recipe is perfect for a quick weeknight meal! The cooked cod will last for up to a day in the fridge - so you may want to make another piece, just to have it available. Serve with sautéed vegetables, a salad, or on top of zucchini noodles for a decadent weeknight dinner!

Serving: 1

Serving Size: 1 piece

Prep Time: 10 minutes

Cook Time: 35 minutes

Ingredients

½ red pepper, diced

1 Tablespoon olive oil

1 teaspoon red pepper flakes

½ lemon, sliced into three equal sized medallions

1 6 oz fillet cod, preferably Ocean Safe certified wild caught

1 teaspoon dried oregano

1 teaspoon dried thyme

1 teaspoon salt

1 teaspoon pepper

Instructions

Preheat the oven to 375F. Toss the pepper with the olive oil and a pinch of salt, and transfer the mixture into an ovenproof baking dish. Bake for 20 minutes, until soft. Transfer the roasted pepper to a blender or food processor, and puree until smooth. Next, lay the cod onto a baking sheet lined with parchment. Preheat oven to 350F. Lay the lemon wheels onto a baking sheet lined with parchment, and place the fish on top. Season the fish with the salt, pepper, thyme, red pepper flakes and oregano, and spoon the pureed pepper over top. Bake 12 minutes. Turn the broiler on to high, and broil for 5 minutes. Serve immediately.

Nutrition: 336 calories, 16.2 g fat, 40 g protein, 6g net carbs

Sea Bass with Prosciutto and Herbs

This recipe is restaurant quality, and so easy to prepare! Eat it on its own for a luxuriously simple dinner, or pair it with zucchini noodles or sautéed spinach.

Serving: 1

Serving Size: 1 piece

Prep Time: 15 minutes

Cook Time: 25 minutes

Ingredients

3 oz sea bass fillet, preferably wild caught

½ lemon, sliced into three equal sized medallions

1 teaspoon dried oregano

1 teaspoon dried thyme

1 teaspoon salt

1 teaspoon pepper

2 Tablespoons olive oil

4 cherry tomatoes

¼ cup basil, chopped finely

3 stalks asparagus

1 Tablespoon butter, melted

1 oz prosciutto, cut into thin ribbons

Instructions

Preheat the oven to 375F. Lay the lemon wheels onto a baking sheet lined with parchment. Brush the fish with 1 Tablespoon of olive oil, and lay it on top of the lemon wheels. Toss the asparagus and tomatoes in the remaining Tablespoon of oil, and arrange it around the fish. Season everything with the salt, pepper and dried herbs. Toss the butter, prosciutto, and basil together, and lay it on top of the fish. Bake for 25 minutes. Serve warm.

Nutrition: 586 calories, 16.2 g fat, 40 g protein, 6g net carbs

Thai Coconut Cod

This fabulously creamy, spicy fish dish goes perfectly on top of cauliflower rice! If you prefer a bit more spice, feel free to add as many chilies as you like; if you're unsure of the heat level, start with one chili - you can always add more at the end! Leftovers keep well for up to two days in the fridge, and can be reheated by microwaving on high for 2 minutes.

Serving: 2

Serving Size: half recipe

Prep Time: 10 minutes

Cook Time: 15 minutes

Ingredients

> 2 6 oz pieces cod
>
> 1 Tablespoon coconut oil
>
> 1/2 can coconut milk
>
> 1 handful cilantro, finely chopped
>
> 8 large basil leaves, chopped
>
> 2 green onions, finely sliced
>
> 1 clove garlic, minced
>
> 1" piece ginger, grated
>
> 4 red chilis, finely sliced (optional)
>
> 1 Tablespoon sesame seeds

For the cauliflower rice:

> ½ cup riced cauliflower
>
> ½ can coconut milk

Instructions

Preheat the oven to 350F. Season the cod with salt and pepper, and lay it onto a baking sheet lined with parchment. Bake in the oven for 20 minutes, until flakey. Meanwhile, drizzle the coconut oil into a small saucepan, and add the green onion, ginger, garlic and chilies. Sauté for 30 seconds, and then add the coconut milk. Taste, and season with salt. Add the cilantro and basil, and reduce heat to low. Simmer 20 minutes. While the cod is in the oven and the coconut sauce is simmering, combine the remaining half can of coconut milk with the cauliflower rice in a microwave safe bowl. Cover, and microwave on high for 4 minutes. Season with salt and pepper, and fluff with a fork. To serve, spoon out the coconut rice onto a plate, and place the fish on top. Spoon the sauce over everything. Garnish with sesame seeds

Nutrition: 482 calories, 34 g fat, 42.5 g protein, 5g net carbs

Thai Coconut Cod Lettuce Wraps

This recipe is perfect for lunch, snacks, or a cold dinner on a hot day! These fabulously portable wraps are the perfect make-ahead thing to pack for a workday lunch or snack, and also make a fun addition to a summer day picnic!

Serving: 1

Serving Size: 3 wraps

Prep Time: 15 minutes

Cook Time: 0 minutes

Ingredients

1 serving Thai Coconut Cod

6 large pieces iceberg lettuce

3 large basil leaves

Handful cilantro, torn

4 red chilis, sliced (optional)

Instructions

Lay the iceberg leaves out two at a time, so they overlap each other slightly. Flake ⅓ of the fish into the first lettuce wrap. Add 1 basil leaf and a few cilantro leaves, as well as the chilies if you're using them. Fold the lettuce around the fish to create a bundle. Secure with a toothpick, or wrap in parchment to keep the wrap secure. Continue on with the next set of ingredients, until all three wraps are finished. Keep in the fridge for up to 24 hours.

Nutrition: 592 calories, 46 g fat, 35 g protein, 6g net carbs

Crab Stuffed Cucumbers

These make an excellent snack, but can also be served as an hors d'oeuvres or a supplemental dish at a brunch or lunch.

Serving: 4

Serving Size: 2 pieces

Prep Time: 15 minutes

Cook Time: 0 minutes

Ingredients

1 cucumber

½ cup cream cheese, softened

2 Tablespoons butter, softened

1 Tablespoon heavy cream

1 teaspoon paprika

1 small handful fresh dill, chopped (plus more for garnish)

¼ cup crab meat, picked through and shredded (canned is fine)

1 teaspoon salt

1 teaspoon pepper

1 lemon, zest only

Instructions

Slice the cucumber into about 8 medallions, each roughly 1 ½" thick. Using a small spoon, carefully scoop out some of the middle, making sure to leave the base intact. Mix together the rest of the ingredients. Spoon the mixture into the cucumber rounds, and garnish with dill. Serve immediately, or keep in an airtight container in the fridge for up to 24 hours.

Nutrition: 179 calories, 17.4 g fat, 3.1 g protein, 3 g net carbs

Salmon with Beurre Blanc

Beurre Blanc is a classic French sauce that is tangy, creamy and deliciously keto friendly! This restaurant quality fish goes beautifully with asparagus or greens. Make sure your chunks of butter are very cold in order to allow the sauce to emulsify properly.

Serving: 4

Serving Size: 1 fillet of fish

Prep Time: 15 minutes

Cook Time: 20 minutes

Ingredients

4 3 oz fillets salmon

2 Tablespoons olive oil

½ lemon, juice and zest

¼ cup dry white wine

¼ cup heavy cream

¼ cup cold butter, cut into chunks

1 Tablespoon fresh dill, chopped

Instructions

Preheat the oven to 350F. Lay the salmon onto a baking sheet lined with parchment paper, and season with salt and pepper. Bake 15 minutes, until the fish is fully cooked. Allow to rest while you prepare the beurre blanc. Preheat a small pan over medium high heat. Add in the wine and lemon juice, and cook until it has almost completely evaporated. Whisk in the cream, and reduce heat to low. Whisk in the cold butter, one chunk at a time, whisking well until it's completely incorporated into the cream. Continue on, until all the butter has been mixed in and a thick, white sauce has formed. Whisk in the dill and lemon zest, and remove the sauce from the heat. Leftovers will keep in an airtight container in the fridge for up to three days.

Nutrition: 330 calories, 28 g fat, 18 g protein, 1g net carbs

Spinach Stuffed Cod

These stuffed cod rolls look fancy, but they're so easy to make and can be rolled in advance for quick heating and serving! Serve them with asparagus, broccoli, peppers or greens!

Serving: 4

Serving Size: 1 fillet of fish

Prep Time: 15 minutes

Cook Time: 25 minutes

Ingredients

> 4 3 oz fillets cod
>
> 1 cup spinach
>
> 1 Tablespoon olive oil
>
> 1 clove garlic, minced
>
> 1 lemon, juice and zest
>
> 1 Tablespoon thyme
>
> 1 teaspoon salt
>
> 1 teaspoon pepper
>
> 4 strips bacon

Instructions

Preheat the oven to 350F. Preheat a medium pan over medium heat. Drizzle in the oil, and add in the garlic, spinach and salt and pepper. Sauté the spinach for a minute or so, and squeeze in the lemon. Continue sautéing until the spinach has wilted down. Set aside. Make an incision into the cod, and slice either side to open up the fillets like a book. Spoon the spinach mixture evenly into the center of each fillet, and fold it back up to cover the filling. Tie a bacon strip around the fillet, to keep it in place. Lay the wrapped fillets onto a baking sheet lined with parchment. Bake 15-20 minutes, until the fish is opaque and flakey. Serve immediately. Leftovers will keep in an airtight container in the fridge for up to three days.

Nutrition: 407 calories, 13.7 g fat, 65.6 g protein, 1g net carbs

Parmesan Crusted Halibut

This parmesan-almond crust is perfect for any type of fish, and also works well on chicken. Halibut is buttery, soft, and really decadent! If you choose to go for a slightly less expensive option, cod makes a great substitute.

Serving: 4

Serving Size: 1 fillet of fish

Prep Time: 15 minutes

Cook Time: 20 minutes

Ingredients

> 4 3 oz fillets halibut
>
> 1 egg, beaten
>
> ¼ cup almond flour
>
> 3 Tablespoons parmesan
>
> 1 teaspoon garlic powder
>
> 1 teaspoon thyme
>
> 1 teaspoon salt
>
> 1 teaspoon pepper
>
> 1 Tablespoon olive oil

Instructions

Preheat the oven to 350F. In a bowl, combine the almond flour, parmesan, garlic, thyme, salt and pepper. Coat each fillet in the egg, and toss into the almond flour mixture. Lay on a baking sheet lined with parchment, and drizzle the oil over top. Bake for 20 minutes. Serve immediately. Leftovers will keep in an airtight container in the fridge for up to three days.

> Nutrition: 266 calories, 14.8 g fat, 30 g protein, 1.2 g net carbs

Crab Stuffed Avocado

This stuffed avocado is creamy and sophisticated! Eat it for a light lunch or dinner, on top of greens.

Serving: 2

Serving Size: ½ avocado

Prep Time: 5 minutes

Cook Time: 0 minutes

Ingredients

> 4 oz crab meat, cooked and picked through
>
> 2 Tablespoons mayonnaise

1 teaspoon salt

1 teaspoon pepper

1 teaspoon paprika

1 avocado, halved

Instructions

Mix together the crab, mayo, and seasonings. Spoon into the avocado halves. Serve immediately.

Nutrition: 319 calories, 25.7 g fat, 9.4 g protein, 6 g net carbs

Fish Tacos

Using leftover Baja Style Halibut Salad, you can easily make these fish tacos for a quick, easy cold lunch! Perfect for a hot day!

Serving: 1

Serving Size: 4 tacos

Prep Time: 5 minutes

Cook Time: 0 minutes

Ingredients

1 serving Baja Style Halibut Salad

8 large pieces iceberg lettuce

2 Tablespoons salsa (optional)

Instructions

Flake the fish and mix with the salad. Lay out 1-2 pieces of lettuce to create a wrap, and spoon ¼ of the mixture into the center. Wrap to form a little taco. Continue until all ingredients have been used. Serve with salsa.

Nutrition: 740 calories, 40 g fat, 95 g protein, 7 g net carbs

Cod Bruschetta

This gorgeous white fish is the perfect vehicle for a combination of tomatoes, prosciutto and herbs! This restaurant quality meal would be great served alongside asparagus or greens.

Serving: 2

Serving Size: 1 fillet

Prep Time: 5 minutes

Cook Time: 25 minutes

Ingredients

2 4 oz pieces cod

1 tomato, diced

½ onion, diced

2 Tablespoons olive oil

1 Tablespoon Italian Herbs

4 oz prosciutto, chopped

Handful fresh parsley, chopped

1 teaspoon salt

1 teaspoon pepper

Instructions

Preheat oven to 350F. Toss together all ingredients, except the fish. Lay the fish onto a baking sheet lined with parchment, and spoon the bruschetta mixture over top. Bake 25 minutes. Serve warm.

Nutrition: 341 calories, 18.2 g fat, 28.4 g protein, 3.5 g net carbs

Desserts and Drinks

Keto Bulletproof Coffee

Boost your coffee's fat content and make your breakfast amazing by enjoying a cup of this delicious Keto friendly Bulletproof Coffee.

Serving: 1

Serving Size:

Prep Time: 5 minutes

Cook Time: 0

Ingredients

1 cup black coffee

1 Tablespoon grass-fed unsalted butter

1 Tablespoon coconut or MCT oil

½ Tablespoon heavy cream

½ teaspoon vanilla extract

Instructions

Mix everything together by hand or in a blender. Serve warm or cold! You can substitute almond extract for the vanilla or leave it out.

Nutrition: 255 calories, 28.5 g fat, 0 g protein, 1.0 g carbohydrates

Almond Butter Bulletproof Coffee

This slightly sweet version of Bulletproof Coffee is a super fast and easy way to get your morning caffeine kick, along with a good dose of fat! Prepared Almond Butter Fat Bombs are added to regular coffee to make this nutty, creamy coffee.

Serving: 1

Serving Size:

Prep Time: 10 minutes

Cook Time: 0

Ingredients

> 1 cup coffee

> 1 Almond Butter Fat Bomb

Instructions

Brew your coffee as you normally would. Using your blender, blend together the coffee and a Fat Bomb. Drink your coffee hot, or add ice cubes for iced coffee.

> Nutrition: 300 calories, 31g fat, 7g protein, 4g net carbs

Chocolate Smoothie

Keto smoothies are having their moment in the spotlight, and it's easy to see why! Creamy, thick and delicious, they are the perfect treat for snacking or breakfast! This chocolate smoothie is so thick and creamy, it'll remind you of a chocolate milkshake! Enjoy it extra cold to really get a satisfying experience!

Servings: 1

Serving Size: whole recipe

Prep Time: 5 minutes

Cook Time: 0 minutes

Ingredients:

> 1 Tablespoon chia seeds

> 1 egg yolk

> 1 Tablespoon almond butter

> 1 Tablespoon cocoa butter

> ¼ cup heavy cream

> 1 Tablespoon cocoa powder

> 1 teaspoon Stevia

> ½ cup ice

1/4 teaspoon chocolate essence (unsweetened) or ¼ teaspoon vanilla extract

Instructions:

Pour the ice and cream into the bottom of the blender, to prevent the other ingredients from sticking to the bottom. Add in the rest of the ingredients, and blend on high until smooth. Serve immediately.

Nutrition: 575 calories, 44 g fat, 34 g protein, 3 g net carbs

Vanilla Smoothie

This creamy vanilla shake is the perfect thing to jump start your day!

Serving: 1

Serving Size: whole recipe

Prep Time: 5 minutes

Cook Time: 0 minutes

Ingredients

    1 cup coconut milk

    1 Tablespoon coconut oil

    ½ Tablespoon vanilla extract

    1 teaspoon Stevia

Instructions

Combine all ingredients in a blender until smooth. Serve immediately.

Nutrition: 669 calories, 70.8g fat, 5.5 g protein, 4 g net carbs

Strawberry Cow Smoothie

This smoothie is refreshing, sweet and fun! When your body adjusts to the keto lifestyle, your taste buds naturally adjust to find foods naturally sweeter. In the beginning, feel free to use a bit of Stevia if you like, but you may find you don't need it!

Serving: 1

Serving Size: whole recipe

Prep Time: 5 minutes

Cook Time: 0 minutes

Ingredients

    ½ cup frozen strawberries

    ½ cup full fat coconut milk

    1 cup ice

Instructions

Pour the coconut milk into the bottom of the blender to prevent the other ingredients from sticking. Add in the rest of the ingredients, and puree until smooth. Serve immediately.

Nutrition: 301 calories, 28.6 g fat, 2.8 g protein, 9 g net carbs

Golden Milk Smoothie

Golden Milk is all the rage these days, and this smoothie is definitely full of benefits! Turmeric has been touted as the newest superfood, and has been proven to cleanse the liver and organs for optimal health. Enjoy this smoothie very cold.

Serving: 1

Serving Size: whole recipe

Prep Time: 5 minutes

Cook Time: 0 minutes

Ingredients

> 1 Tablespoon turmeric
>
> 1 cup coconut milk
>
> 1 teaspoon Stevia
>
> 1 cup crushed ice

Instructions

Puree all ingredients together until smooth. Serve immediately.

Nutrition: 460 calories, 25.3 g fat, 1.7g protein, 1.4 g net carbs

Almond Butter Smoothie

This is a filling and yummy smoothie you can have for breakfast or as a quick snack to up your fat intake. It's super low carb and delicious!

Serving: 2

Serving Size: about 1 cup

Prep Time: 5 minutes

Cook Time: 0 minutes

Ingredients

> 2 Tablespoons almond butter
>
> 1 1/2 cups almond milk
>
> 1 Tablespoon hemp seeds

Instructions

Start by pouring the almond milk into the blender to avoid the ingredients sticking at the bottom. Add in the rest of the ingredients. Turn the blender on, starting at a low speed and increase as needed. Add extra water if you desire your smoothie more on the liquid side. Pour into a cup and serve immediately. Place any leftover smoothie into an airtight container, and enjoy within 24 hours.

Nutrition: 483 calories, 34.6g fat, 5.5g protein, 4g net carbs

Pink Power Smoothie

This smoothie is full of good fat, and a great flavor and color! Keep any leftovers in an airtight container in the fridge for up to 24 hours so you can enjoy a quick pick me up later on!

Serving: 2

Serving Size: half recipe

Prep Time: 5 minutes

Cook Time: 0 minutes

Ingredients

> 1/2 cup raspberries
>
> 1/2 Tablespoon lemon zest
>
> 1 cup coconut milk
>
> 1 Tablespoon flaxseeds

Instructions

Start by pouring the coconut milk into the blender to avoid the ingredients sticking at the bottom. Add in the rest of the ingredients. Turn the blender on, starting at a low speed and increase as needed. Add extra water if you desire your smoothie more on the liquid side. Once it looks even, pour into a cup and serve immediately. Pour any leftover smoothie into an airtight container and enjoy within 24 hours.

Nutrition: 310 calories, 29.9g fat, 3.8g protein, 9g net carbs

Raspberry Chia Pudding

Chia pudding is so versatile, and really easy to prep in advance! Because chia seeds get better as they expand in liquid, this pudding will continue to thicken and sweeten as it sits in the fridge. The best part is, it's good for up to a week in the fridge, so if you're a really big fan of it you can make enough to last you all week, and indulge as needed.

Serving: 2

Serving Size: about 3/4 cup

Prep Time: 5 minutes

Cook Time: 5 minutes

Ingredients

1 cup almond milk

1/2 cup chia seeds

¼ cup frozen raspberries

1 Tablespoon flaxseeds

1 Tablespoon hemp seeds

Instructions

Combine all ingredients together, mixing well so the raspberries crush a bit. Store in an airtight container overnight. Enjoy leftovers within 7 days.

Nutrition: 642 calories, 50 g fat, 15.9 g protein, 8g net carbs

Raspberry Chocolate Fudge

This rich, chocolaty fudge is the perfect thing to hit the spot when you're craving something sweet. Best of all, it's virtually carb and protein free and high fat, which can help kick start your ketosis.

Serving: 16

Serving Size: 1 piece

Prep Time: 2 minutes

Cook Time: 10 Minutes

Ingredients

½ cup raw cacao powder

2 Tablespoons unsweetened dark chocolate, shaved

2 Tablespoons Stevia

½ cup coconut oil

¼ cup raspberries, mashed lightly

¼ cup almond milk

Instructions

Mix all ingredients together until well combined. Prepare a 10" baking dish with parchment paper or plastic wrap, and carefully spoon the fudge mixture into the center. Using a spatula, spread the mixture evenly into the baking dish, and cover with plastic wrap. Refrigerate for an hour, and cut into 16 equal pieces. Store wrapped in the fridge for up to one month.

Nutrition: 74 calories, 8.1g fat, 0.6g protein, 0.9g net carbs

Strawberry Chia Pudding Popsicles

Popsicles are such a sweet, refreshing treat! These popsicles have extra fat and protein from coconut milk and chia seeds, and are sweetened naturally with fruit (although you can use a bit of Stevia if you like).

Serving: 6

Serving Size: 1 popsicle

Prep Time: 4 hours, including freezing time

Cook Time: 0 minutes

Ingredients

2 cups coconut milk

¼ cup chia seeds

¼ cup frozen strawberries, thawed

Instructions

Mash together the berries and chia seeds. Stir in the coconut milk. Transfer the mixture to 6 popsicle molds, and freeze for at least 4 hours. Popsicles will last in the freezer for up to 8 weeks.

Nutrition: 277 calories, 24.9 g fat, 5 g protein, 3 g net carbs

Almond Butter Cookies

These cookies are reminiscent of childhood – soft and chewy – while staying extremely low carb and high fat! What more could you want?

Servings: 10

Serving Size: 1 cookie

Prep Time: 5 minutes

Cook Time: 10 minutes

Ingredients:

¾ cup almond butter

¼ cup powdered Stevia or erythritol

1 egg yolk

¼ teaspoon cinnamon

Instructions:

Preheat oven to 350F. In a medium sized bowl, beat together all ingredients until smooth. Roll the cookie dough into 1-1 ½" balls, and lay them out onto a baking sheet lined with parchment. Press each ball down with a fork, to form the final cookie shape. Bake 10-12 minutes, until golden brown and fragrant. Let the cookies cool completely before serving. Store cookies in an airtight container at room temperature for up to a week.

Nutrition: 98 calories, 10 g fat, 4 g protein, 1.4 g net carbs

Snacks and Sides

Butter Tossed Asparagus

The old adage is true - butter DOES make it better! This asparagus dish is loaded with delicious fat and flavor and makes the perfect side dish.

Servings: 2

Serving Size: 5 pieces

Prep Time: 0 minutes

Cook Time: 15 minutes

Ingredients:

> 10 spears fresh asparagus
>
> 2 Tablespoons butter
>
> 1 Tablespoon olive oil
>
> 2 large stems thyme
>
> 1 teaspoon salt
>
> 1 teaspoon white pepper

Instructions:

Bring a large pot of salted water to a boil. Toss in the asparagus spears, and boil for 1 minute to blanch. Drain, and transfer to an ice bath. Set aside. Preheat a large pan over medium heat. Drizzle in the oil and add the butter and whole thyme stem. Cook until the butter has melted fully and has started to foam, about 2 minutes. Add the blanched asparagus spears to the foaming butter, and toss well to coat. Cook for 1-2 minutes, tossing well the entire time. Serve immediately.

> Nutrition: 186 calories, 18.7 g fat, 2.8 g protein, 2 g net carbs

Caramelized Onions

These caramelized onions are low carb, relatively high fat, and make a great addition to pizzas, burgers, or anything else you can come up with.

Servings: 8

Serving Size: 1 Tablespoon

Prep Time: 10 minutes

Cook Time: 65 minutes

Ingredients:

> 4 onions, sliced thinly
>
> ½ lb butter

1 Tablespoon salt

Instructions:

Melt the butter in a pan over medium heat. Add in the onions and the salt. Toss well with tongs until the onions start to cook down. Continue to cook, stirring occasionally, for about an hour, until the onions are brown and soft. Transfer to an airtight container and keep in the fridge for up to 4 weeks.

Nutrition: 225 calories, 23.1 g fat, 0.9 g protein, 3 g net carbs

Curry Mayonnaise

Curry Mayo is a great option to mix up flavors! Use this mayo on burgers or in the Egg Salad or Chicken Salad as a substitute.

Servings: 8

Serving Size: 1 Tablespoon

Prep Time: 5 minutes

Cook Time: 0 minutes

Ingredients:

¼ cup mayonnaise

1 Tablespoon curry powder

Instructions:

Whisk ingredients together until smooth. Store in an airtight container for up to 5 weeks.

Nutrition: 45 calories, 5 g fat, 0 g protein, 0 g net carbs

Green Tahini

This tahini is enhanced with greens for additional nutritional value and a hit of color! Use this sauce as a dip for veggies, a dressing for salads, or as a replacement for mayo.

Servings: 8

Serving Size: 1 Tablespoon

Prep Time: 5 minutes

Cook Time: 0 minutes

Ingredients:

2 Tablespoons tahini paste

2 cloves garlic

2 teaspoons salt

1 Tablespoon olive oil

1 lemon, juice and zest

¼ cup water

¼ cup fresh kale

Instructions:

In a blender or food processor, combine all ingredients until smooth. Taste and adjust seasoning as needed. Store in an airtight container for up to a month.

Nutrition: 43 calories, 3.9 g fat, 0.7 g protein, 0.3 g net carbs

Cheesy Fondue

Fondue is one of the best snacks for sharing. By using low carb veggies like celery and red peppers, you (and your friends!) can enjoy this high fat, low carb treat.

Serving: 4

Serving Size: 2 pieces pickles, 2 pieces pepper, 3 pieces celery, ¼ fondue sauce

Prep Time: 10 minutes

Cook Time: 30 Minutes

Ingredients

1 cup cheddar cheese, shredded

1 cup gruyere cheese, shredded

¼ cup dry white wine

1 cup heavy cream

1 teaspoon garlic powder

1 teaspoon salt

1 teaspoon cayenne (optional)

3 stalks celery, chopped into 12 equal sticks

½ red bell pepper, sliced into 8 thin strips

4 pickles, cut in half lengthwise

Instructions:

In a medium sized saucepan, melt the cheeses and wine together over medium heat. Stir in the cream and spices, mixing well to combine. Transfer the finished sauce to a fondue pot, and keep warm. Arrange the veggies and bread onto a plate. Using fondue forks, dip the veggies into the cheese sauce and eat immediately.

Nutrition: 376 calories, 32 g fat, 19.5g protein, 4.4 g net carbs

Green Bean Fries

Have a craving for fries, but no potatoes on the Keto Diet, so what do you do? Try these delicious green bean fries smothered in a cheesy herbed mixture. Yummy!

Serving: 4

Serving Size: 8 Pieces

Prep Time: 10 minutes

Cook Time: 10 Minutes

Ingredients

> 24 green beans
>
> 1 egg
>
> ½ cup parmesan
>
> 1 teaspoon garlic powder
>
> 1 teaspoon Italian herbs
>
> 1 teaspoon salt

Instructions

Preheat oven to 400F. Fill a small pot with water up to three quarters. Bring the water to a boil. Blanch the beans for 2 minutes, and immediately drain and transfer them to an ice bath. Next, beat the egg in one bowl, and combine the dry ingredients in another bowl. Prepare a baking sheet lined with parchment. Bread each bean by dipping it first into the egg, then into the cheese mixture. Lay the prepared beans on the baking sheet, and bake for 15 minutes until crispy. Store any leftover beans in an airtight container at room temperature, and enjoy within 4 days.

> Nutrition: 113 calories, 6g fat, 9g protein, 2g net carbs

Seed Crackers & Guacamole

This excellent seed cracker recipe is delicious and makes a perfect snack! You can also have these crackers with soup, as a snack, or to put in a work lunch.

Serving: 4

Serving Size: About 3 crackers, with 2 Tablespoons guac

Prep Time: 10 minutes

Cook Time: 45 Minutes

Ingredients

> 1/4 cup chia seeds
>
> 1/4 cups sesame seeds
>
> 1/4 cups sunflower seeds
>
> 1/2 Tablespoon Italian herbs

1/2 teaspoon salt

1 cup water

1 egg

1/2 mashed avocado

Juice of half a lime

Pinch of sea salt

Instructions

Preheat the oven to 350F. Combine the seeds, herbs, salt and egg in a bowl, and allow the mixture to sit for 5 minutes. Line a baking sheet with parchment paper and spread the seed mixture evenly until flat. Bake for 30 minutes. While still warm, cut the seed mixture into 12 equal sized squares. Flip the crackers over, and bake for another 15 minutes. While the crackers are baking combine all the guacamole ingredients in a bowl and mash until smooth.

Nutrition: 280 calories, 24g fat, 8g protein, 3g net carbs

Celery and Almond Butter

There are many wonderful flavors and textures in this simple and easy snack! The crispy green crunch of celery pairs perfectly with creamy nutty almond butter.

Serving: 1

Serving Size: 8 pieces celery, 2 Tbsp almond butter

Prep Time: 2 minutes

Cook Time: 0 Minutes

Ingredients

2 stalks celery

2 Tablespoons almond butter

Instructions

Cut the celery into 8 equal sized sticks and dip into the almond butter. For a more portable snack, spread the almond butter into the cavity of the celery stalk, and pack in an airtight container for up to 24 hours.

Nutrition: 230 calories, 18g fat, 8g protein, 4g net carbs

Salted Macadamias

Nuts are a great way to get a quick dose of fat. These nuts are SO easy to do, and so delicious! Once you've figured out the basic recipe, it's easy to season these nuts with any herbs or spices.

Serving: 1

Serving Size: whole recipe

Prep Time: 5 minutes

Cook Time: 5 Minutes

Ingredients

1/4 cup Macadamia nuts

1 Tablespoon coconut oil

1 teaspoon sea salt

Instructions

Preheat oven to 350F. Toss the macadamia nuts in the oil and salt. Lay onto a baking sheet, and bake 5 minutes, making sure not to burn the nuts. Allow to cool fully.

Nutrition: 224 calories, 22g fat, 3g protein, 1g net carbs

Nordic Seed Bread

This bread is said to have been invented by the Vikings, and has recently gained new popularity. This variation uses flax, pumpkin seeds, walnuts, macadamia nuts, and almonds. You can swap out the nuts or change the proportions according to your taste; just avoid higher carb nuts like cashews and pistachios.

Servings: 12

Serving Size: 1 piece

Prep Time: 10 minutes

Cook Time: 30 minutes

Ingredients:

1 cup almonds

1 cup walnuts

1 cup ground flax seeds

1 cup pumpkin seeds

1 cup sesame seeds

½ cup ground macadamia nuts

½ cup sesame seeds

5 eggs

½ cup coconut oil

2 teaspoons salt

Instructions:

Preheat oven to 325F. In a large bowl, whisk together the eggs, oil and salt. Add in the seeds, and mix well to combine. Next, press the mixture into a loaf pan lined with parchment. Bake for 1 hour, and allow to cool fully before slicing. Slice the bread into 12 equal sized pieces, and wrap individually. Keep leftover pieces individually wrapped at room temperature for up to 4 weeks.

Nutrition: 369 calories, 31.5 g fat, 10 g protein, 5 g net carbs

Almond Butter Fat Bombs

With a nutty flavor and lots of good fats, these Fat Bombs are one bite snacks you'll really enjoy. You'll need mini muffin tins or muffin cups to make these!

Servings: 6

Serving Size: 1 Fat Bomb

Prep Time: 5 minutes

Cook Time: 5 minutes

Ingredients:

¼ cup almond butter

¼ cup coconut oil

2 Tablespoons cocoa powder

¼ cup Stevia or erythritol

Instructions:

With a mixer or by hand, mix together the almond butter and a coconut oil. Microwave for about 30-45 seconds to soften, then stir until smooth. Add the cocoa powder and the sweetener, then stir those in and mix well. Pour into either silicone or mini muffin tins lined with papers. Stick in the fridge until firm.

Nutrition: 189 calories, 19.1 g fat, 3.2 g protein, 1.4 g net carbs

Mediterranean Fat Bombs

Most Fat Bombs focus on sweet - these are definitely savory and also have a high salt content to help replenish any lost electrolytes.

Servings: 6

Serving Size: 1 piece

Prep Time: 10 minutes

Cook Time: 5 minutes

Ingredients:

½ cup cream cheese

¼ cup butter

1 teaspoon dried oregano

1 teaspoon dried thyme

1 teaspoon dried basil

1 teaspoon garlic powder

5 pieces of sundried tomatoes, sliced

3 olives, sliced

¼ cup parmesan cheese, grated

½ teaspoon salt

1 teaspoon pepper

Instructions:

Beat together the butter and cream cheese until smooth. Beat in the rest of the ingredients, making sure everything is evenly mixed. Prepare a baking dish with a bit of coconut oil. Spoon the mixture in, and spread it evenly throughout the dish. Refrigerate for an hour, up to 6 weeks. Cut into 6 equal pieces.

Nutrition: 155 calories, 15 g fat, 3 g protein, 1.2 g net carbs

Tahini Sauce

Tahini Sauce is a flavor-packed sauce made with sesame paste (also known as tahini). This thick, creamy, dairy free sauce is the perfect dip for veggies, but can also be used as a dressing in lettuce wraps, a sauce for meat, or salad dressing! Double or even quadruple the tahini recipe and keep some on hand in the fridge to use as needed- it will easily last for up to two weeks in an airtight container!

Servings: 1

Serving Size: 20 veggie sticks, with about ¼ cup tahini

Prep Time: 10 minutes

Cook Time: 0 minutes

Ingredients:

1 Tablespoon tahini paste

1 teaspoon chopped parsley

1 Tablespoon lemon juice

¼ cup water

½ Tablespoon salt

1 clove garlic

¼ cup olive oil

½ cucumber, cut into 8 equal pieces

1 stalk celery, cut into 8 equal pieces

Instructions:

In a blender or food processor, combine the tahini, parsley, lemon juice, water, salt, garlic and oil until smooth. Transfer to an airtight container, and store in the fridge for up to two weeks. Serve with veggie sticks.

Nutrition: 555 calories, 58.5 g fat, 4 g protein, 8 g net carbs

Baked Brie

This baked Brie recipe is savory, comforting, and nice for special occasions. For added decadence, serve with Nordic seed bread and sliced low carb veggies like celery, cucumber, or peppers.

Servings: 2

Serving Size: ½ wheel

Prep Time: 5 minutes

Cook Time: 10 minutes

Ingredients:

> 6 oz Brie cheese
>
> ½ oz walnuts
>
> ½ oz pine nuts
>
> ½ oz pecans
>
> 1 clove garlic, minced
>
> 2 teaspoons smoked paprika
>
> 4 stems thyme
>
> 1 Tablespoon salt
>
> 1 Tablespoon pepper
>
> 1 Tablespoon olive oil

Instructions:

Preheat the oven to 375F. In a medium sized bowl, combine the nuts, garlic, herbs, paprika, salt, pepper and oil. Lay the cheese onto a baking sheet lined with parchment, and spoon the nut mixture over top, so it completely covers the cheese. Bake for 10 minutes, until the cheese is melted and the nuts are fragrant and toasted. Any unfinished cheese can be wrapped and kept in the fridge for up to a month.

Nutrition: 501 calories, 44 g fat, 21 g protein, 3.4 g net carbs

Spicy Mayo

This spicy mayo makes a wonderful burger topper, and is also a great dip for veggies, fried pickles, onion rings, or anything else you can think of! Make a big batch and keep in the fridge!

Servings: 12

Serving Size: 2 Tablespoons

Prep Time: 10 minutes

Cook Time: 10 minutes

Ingredients:

   3 cups mayonnaise

   6 Tablespoons hot sauce or sriracha

Instructions:

Whisk the two ingredients together until smooth. Keep in the fridge for up to 8 weeks.

   Nutrition: 90 calories, 10 g fat, 0 g protein, 0 g net carbs

Chapter 9:
Keto Tips and FAQs

In the previous two chapters, you received two separate 4-week meal plans, plus 100 recipes to get you started on the Keto Diet. But I want to make sure I've covered absolutely everything in this book, so in this chapter, I'm going to answer some frequently asked questions, as well as supplying you with even more tips and tricks to sustain the Keto Lifestyle long term. Let's get started!

Keto Diet FAQ

Q: Is It Okay to Be in Ketosis for a Long Time, Like Two Years or Longer?

A: Yes! While being in a state of ketosis was originally designed to see our human ancestors through annual six-month winters with limited food resources, there is absolutely no medical or scientific evidence to back up the claim that long term ketosis is harmful for the body in any way. It is a restrictive diet that may be difficult mentally to keep up long term, but it doesn't have any physical long term negative side effects. Get regular medical check-ups at least every six to eight months. Monitor your blood and breath using Keto Monitors. You'll be just fine!

Q: Is It Okay to Cycle In and Out of Ketosis?

A: Yes, it is! As stated previously, our human ancestors would usually go into a ketosis metabolic state every single winter. You don't want your insulin levels to get too low. You can incorporate intermittent fasting as part of the Keto Diet as well. To cycle out of ketosis, gradually increase your carbohydrate count. The only downside to cycling in and out of ketosis is that you'll experience Keto Flu type symptoms each time you go back into ketosis. But it's fine to kick yourself out of ketosis for a period of time. Don't be surprised if you don't feel good or gain some weight back, though! Being out of ketosis comes with its own side effects.

Q: How Can I Be a Vegetarian and Go Keto at the Same Time?

A: Just because you're vegetarian doesn't mean you should find the Keto Diet too restrictive and not try it. You'll still follow your Macros, but you'll get your protein predominantly from nuts, eggs, and dairy items. Other sources include vegetarian 'meat' sources like tempeh, tofu, and seitan. You'll also need to take supplements, like Vitamins D3, DHA & EPA, and the minerals of iron and zinc. You will need to watch your carbs as a vegetarian, because it can be tempting to eat too many. Eat lots of good low-carb veggies, especially spinach, kale, broccoli, cauliflower, and zucchini. Also, consume plenty of plant based oils, especially coconut oil, MCT oil, olive oil, avocado oil, and red palm oil. There are plenty of vegan 'dairy' options you can purchase as well. Read your food labels and purchase the products that have the most proteins and good fats.

Q: How Long Before I See Better Health and Weight Loss?

A: Within the first month! The quicker you can get into ketosis, the quicker you'll see better health and weight loss. For some people, jumping in feet first is a welcome challenge. They'll start the meal plan, get cooking, and start feeling the effects within a few days. But for most of us, easing into such a restrictive diet takes a little more time. The longer you're in ketosis, the more benefits you'll experience.

Q: Will There Be Kidney Stones on the Keto Diet?

A: Your liver gets all the credit for producing ketones, but your kidneys play an important role in this diet, too. Your body is 70% water, so you really do need to stay ultra hydrated on this diet. If you don't, that increases the amount of uric acid in your body, producing kidney stones and gout. Remember, this is not Atkins! It's a medium protein diet, not a high protein diet. The fats are really what you want to be consuming. Follow the meal plan guidelines in the previous chapters and balance your good fats. Drink lots of water with lemon in it. The citrates in lemon keep calcium molecules from sticking together, thus preventing kidney stones. If you're still concerned, take oral potassium citrate tablets to decrease the likelihood of kidney stones.

Q: Why Am I Losing Muscle On This Diet?

A: Your muscles are one of the places on your body where extra glycogen is stored. So, when you switch to a very low carb diet, within a few days your body starts searching for any leftover glycogen to be used as energy. That's why you start losing muscle. After just four weeks of being in ketosis on the diet, your muscle glycogen counts will drop to about half. This makes sense from a historical standpoint, too; when your human ancestors went into ketosis in the winter, that was to conserve muscle energy, not expend it. This diet is excellent for those looking to lose weight and overcome a number of ailments. But if you're seeking a high intensity workout or are an athlete, then consult a nutritionist to keep your muscles in peak physical condition.

Tips for Ketogenic Diet Success!

Up until now, you've read dozens of tips and tricks on how to change your eating habits to the Keto Diet lifestyle! You've cleaned out your cupboards and replaced carbohydrates with plenty of good fats. You've started on a meal plan, learned to cook new recipes, and transitioned after the first four weeks.

But in order to have success on the Keto Diet for a long time, we've got some more helpful information for you.

Keto Diet on a Wallet Diet

How do you both save money and save carbohydrates while staying in ketosis? There are many ways to stick to a financial budget. One tip is to purchase your pantry items in bulk. You can keep a price book to compare the prices in stores between things like olive oil, nuts and seeds, chicken broth, and baking ingredients. Purchase large food storage containers to store your bulk purchases in your pantry.

Shop around at different stores. You can find inexpensive herbs, spices, and vegetables at ethnic markets. Things like coconut milk, curry pastes, soy sauce, teriyaki sauce, and a huge fish selection are at Asian markets. Their prices are usually much lower than American supermarkets. Don't forget to compare online prices, too. You could score amazing deals off Amazon.com.

Your freezer can also help you save money. Buy meats or fish in bulk, then individually package them in plastic bags and store in the freezer. You can put butter in the freezer, too!

Buy generic store brands instead of national brands, which spend millions of dollars a year on marketing. Generic canned tomatoes, frozen vegetables, and baking items are much less expensive.

Fall Back Keto Foods

Yep, we all get tired in the evening and just want to whip up a quick batch of pasta and sauce. It's so easy … and it's not Keto friendly. Always have Keto safe fall back foods to keep in the back of your mind, for the times you're too tired and your blood sugar is too low to think.

Try these ones:

- Hard boiled eggs
- Cottage cheese
- Nuts or seeds
- Slice of cheese
- Keto Fat Bomb
- Easy smoothie

Meal Prepping

You want to know the real secret to cooking fast, easy meals? Take care of the meal prep beforehand! You can marinate meats, slice or dice veggies, defrost foods, and put together dry baking mixes before you do your actual cooking. I keep plastic containers of cooked shredded chicken, sliced celery, and diced onions in my fridge. I eat those three foods all the time. That way, it's easy to throw together a quick salad or soup. Choose the foods that you eat frequently, and prepare them to keep in your fridge or pantry. That makes cooking much faster.

Family Keto Fun

How about converting your family to also eat on the Keto Diet with you? It's much easier to not eat any bread when nobody in the house is eating it, either. It also cuts down on meal preparation time, since you're not making two dishes. For kids, you can turn it into a game to see what foods they can eat, too. The Ketogenic Diet works whether you are single or you have a family. When you have a family situation, then here are tips to make the transition:

- Sit down with your family members and tell them the new diet you're going to be on
- Have everyone together, as a family, decide on the meals that look good from those provided in this book
- Create a new grocery list based on those meals and shop for those ingredients with family members
- Try out these new meals and recipes, starting with easy ones pretty much everyone loves (omelets, burgers, salads, etc.)

Jump Around

Getting some sort of daily movement or exercise into your schedule will only help your body along your Keto Diet journey. It's excellent to see your weight loss, and the tendency is to just leave it and enjoy that natural weight loss. But you are a human being that was designed to walk and enjoy all the benefits of daily moving around. There are many places to start a simple walking routine: in nature, in a city downtown, inside a shopping mall or galleria, or in neighborhoods.

Put Together a Recipe Collection

Get some more recipe books! For those of you on a budget, you can get a library card and read the cookbooks. You can also buy used books online at Amazon.com or Barnes and Noble. There are many helpful Keto Dieters on the internet who share their experiences and their recipes, too. Put together your own collection, with your own cooking notes. It will give you a much greater variety and help you explore more of what this diet is all about.

Show Off Your Progress

One of the best things about eating the Keto Diet is you'll physically see such a change in your body. I encourage you to celebrate and show off your progress! Post your pictures on social media, treat yourself to new clothes, and reward your hard work with (non-food) items that bring you joy.

You'll be much happier and have more energy to enjoy and do the things you want with the people you love.

Conclusion:
Your Food, Your Health

In many ways for me, this Ketogenic Diet book has been part instruction manual and part memoir. I've shared with you my personal health challenges that brought me to this diet many years ago.

It's meant a lot to me to see and experience the changes in my own life that have come from a healthier body. It helped my issues with diabetes, which honestly scared me. I don't have any fear about health issues anymore. That's an extraordinary reward that the Keto Diet has bestowed on me. How would you like to be that way, too?

To Be Read Again and Again

There's plenty of books out there you'll read to the last page, put down, and never pick up again. That's not what this book is designed for. It's a guide and a manual for you to read over and over. Reread the chapters on Macros, benefits, and troubleshooting. Really think about the meal plans and the recipes. Pay attention to the bevy of amazing tips and tricks sprinkled throughout the previous pages.

This book is excellent for those who are just starting out and have barely heard of the Keto Diet. It will help you. It's also designed for Keto Dieters who are having issues getting what they want out of the diet, whether that's weight loss or health. I'm very proud of my 30-minute fast meal plan, because I'm super busy myself and knew others are, too. And finally, I wrote this so that the Keto Diet doesn't become just another nutritional fad project in your life. But that it takes root and grows as its own part of your lifestyle, sustaining itself and giving you plenty of rewards and benefits along the way.

What you eat is so important. You don't need a health scare to tell you how important; you know it already.

So, let's eat the good stuff your body can use for a different form of energy. One that will give so much back to you every day of your life!

Might sound like a repeat tooting but hey, sometimes we all just need a little reminder right?

If you have taken away 1 single useful thing of value or learnt something that you thought was nice and helpful, could you please help a friend out and leave a review over in amazon?

It's totally great that you are sharing with folks about the book and this will then help more folks to know about what you know too!

Thank you so much!

Appendix

Grocery List for Each Meal Plan

Here is a grocery list for you! It's split into two-week lists, so that you only have to shop every other weekend. You also get grocery lists for both meal plans. Buying in bulk saves you time and money, so do that whenever you can.

Before we get started with the lists, you'll want to stock your pantry with Keto approved ingredients. These form the basis for almost every recipe! Every two weeks, you'll go through the following list and make sure you have enough. If not, add the restocked item to the grocery list:

Restock the Pantry Every Two Weeks with the Following:

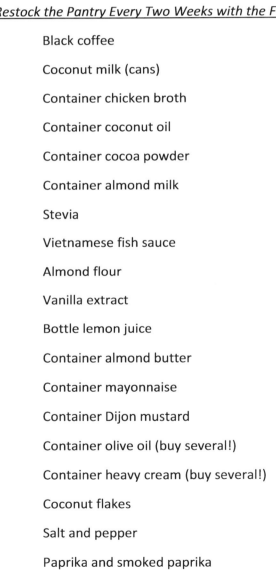

Black coffee

Coconut milk (cans)

Container chicken broth

Container coconut oil

Container cocoa powder

Container almond milk

Stevia

Vietnamese fish sauce

Almond flour

Vanilla extract

Bottle lemon juice

Container almond butter

Container mayonnaise

Container Dijon mustard

Container olive oil (buy several!)

Container heavy cream (buy several!)

Coconut flakes

Salt and pepper

Paprika and smoked paprika

Cinnamon

Ground cumin

Cayenne pepper (dried)

Chili powder

Italian herbs

Oregano

Thyme

Nutmeg

Ginger

Allspice

Turmeric

Garam Masala

Garlic powder

Onion powder

Fennel seed

Ground coriander (cilantro)

Chopped pecans

Almonds

Walnuts

Macadamia nuts

Ground flax seeds

Pumpkin seeds

Sesame seeds

Sunflower seeds

Hemp seeds

Chia seeds

Basic Meal Plan Grocery List:

First 2 Weeks:

Produce & Fresh Herbs:

7 avocados

5 green bell peppers

2 red bell peppers

3 limes

6 lemons

3 bunches celery

Container cherry tomatoes

6 tomatoes

36 green beans

Package shiitake mushrooms

Package cremini mushrooms

3 red onions

6 yellow onions

2 radishes

2 cucumbers

2 heads Romaine lettuce

2 heads iceberg lettuce

2 heads kale

1 bunch arugula

Fresh cilantro, parsley, basil, and dill

4 jalapenos

2 Scotch bonnets

1 bunch green onions

1 package bean sprouts

1 small carrot

Fresh spinach

Garlic cloves

1 leek

10 spears asparagus

2 zucchinis

1 head broccoli

3 heads cauliflower

Jar of artichoke hearts

Jar green olives

Jar sundried tomatoes

Small package raspberries

Meat & Seafood:

1 lb steak

1 lb ground pork

8 lbs ground beef

1 lb ground lamb

2 6 oz lamb chops

2 4 oz pieces salmon

2 packages bacon

6 shrimp

4 3 oz cod fillets

2 4 ounce pieces of halibut

1 8 oz ahi tuna steak

1 whole chicken

8 large chicken breasts

3 lbs boneless chicken thighs

4 pork chops

Package prosciutto

2 ounces salami

Eggs & Dairy:

3 one dozen egg cartons

3 packages butter

Package gruyere

Package shredded parmesan

Package shredded cheddar

Package block cream cheese

Container plain Greek yogurt

6 oz goat cheese

Other:

2 14.5 ounce cans crushed tomatoes

Jar salsa

Jar dill pickles

Package frozen strawberries

Package frozen raspberries

Container avocado oil

Bottle sesame oil

MCT oil

White wine vinegar

1 bar unsweetened dark chocolate

Thai red/yellow/green curry paste

Bottle white wine

Second 2 Weeks:

Produce & Fresh Herbs:

9 avocados

3 green bell peppers

1 red pepper

2 lemons

7 limes

Container cherry tomatoes

5 regular tomatoes

Garlic cloves

3 red onions

5 yellow onions

1 bunch green onions

24 green beans

1 jalapeno

2 Scotch bonnets

8 red Thai chilis

Fresh basil, dill, cilantro, and parsley

Package white mushrooms

Package cremini mushrooms

3 asparagus stalks

5 zucchinis

1 cucumber

1 carrot

2 bunches celery

Bunch arugula

1 head iceberg lettuce

2 heads kale

1 head Romaine lettuce

1 leek

2 heads broccoli

3 heads cauliflower

Small package raspberries

Meat & Seafood:

4 lbs flank steak

1 lb skirt steak

1 lb ground beef

2 lbs smoked salmon

½ lb ham

1 cup ground pork rinds

Large package bacon

1 oz prosciutto

2 6 oz pieces cod

4 3 oz halibut fillets

3 oz fillet of sea bass

½ lb white fish

9 scallops

¼ lb shrimp

¼ lb crab meat

4 chicken thighs, bone in skin on

13 large chicken breasts, boneless, skinless

Eggs & Dairy:

4 one dozen egg cartons

4 packages butter

Gruyere

Package block cream cheese

Package shredded mozzarella

Package shredded cheddar

Package shredded Parmesan

Package shredded Monterey Jack cheese

2 lbs goat cheese

Other:

Bottle white wine

Bottle red wine

Package frozen strawberries

Package frozen raspberries

Bottle avocado oil

Bottle sesame oil

White wine vinegar

Red/yellow/green curry paste

Container beef stock or broth

1 14.5 oz can diced tomatoes

2 14.5 oz cans crushed tomatoes

Bottle Worcestershire sauce

Jar tahini paste

Jar salsa

Soy sauce

Cocoa butter

Bottle of hot sauce or sriracha

30-Minute Fast Meals Grocery List:

First 2 Weeks:

Produce & Fresh Herbs:

7 avocados

Package cherry tomatoes

7 regular tomatoes

2 red onions

4 yellow onions

4 green bell peppers

2 red bell peppers

2 radishes

6 lemons

3 limes

3 jalapenos

4 Thai red chilis

Garlic cloves

2 bunches green onions

Package white mushrooms

2 packages cremini mushrooms

Package shiitake mushrooms

1 package bean sprouts

Fresh basil, dill, cilantro, and parsley

Package fresh raspberries

10 green beans

2 zucchinis

2 cucumbers

1 carrot

2 bunches celery

3 heads Romaine lettuce

1 head iceberg lettuce

3 bunches kale

1 bunch arugula

3 heads broccoli

2 heads cauliflower

Meat & Seafood:

2 lbs ground beef

1 lb ground pork

1 lb ground lamb

1 lb steak

1 lb skirt steak

1 lb flank steak

2 6 oz lamb chops

4 oz smoked salmon

4 4 oz cod fillets

4 4oz pieces of halibut

2 4 oz salmon pieces

1 8 oz ahi tuna steak

6 shrimp

6 slices bacon

6 oz prosciutto

2 oz salami

6 large chicken breasts, boneless skinless

Eggs & Dairy:

2 one dozen egg cartons

5 packages stick butter

Package shredded mozzarella

Package shredded parmesan

2 packages block cream cheese

Container Greek yogurt

Other:

Package frozen strawberries

2 packages frozen raspberries

Jar sundried tomatoes

Jar green olives

Jar artichoke hearts

Container tahini paste

Bottle sesame oil

Cocoa butter

Bottle fish sauce

Cacao powder

Soy sauce

Second 2 Weeks:

Produce & Fresh Herbs:

7 avocados

Package cherry tomatoes

7 regular tomatoes

2 red onions

4 yellow onions

4 green bell peppers

2 red bell peppers

2 radishes

6 lemons

3 limes

3 jalapenos

4 Thai red chilis

Garlic cloves

2 bunches green onions

Package white mushrooms

2 packages cremini mushrooms

Package shiitake mushrooms

1 package bean sprouts

Fresh basil, dill, cilantro, and parsley

Package fresh raspberries

30 green beans

2 zucchinis

2 cucumbers

1 carrot

2 bunches celery

3 heads Romaine lettuce

1 head iceberg lettuce

3 bunches kale

1 bunch arugula

3 heads broccoli

2 heads cauliflower

Meat & Seafood:

2 lbs ground beef

1 lb ground pork

1 lb ground lamb

1 lb steak

1 lb skirt steak

1 lb flank steak

2 6 oz lamb chops

4 oz smoked salmon

4 4 oz cod fillets

4 4oz pieces of halibut

2 4 oz salmon pieces

1 8 oz ahi tuna steak

6 shrimp

6 slices bacon

6 oz prosciutto

2 oz salami

6 large chicken breasts, boneless skinless

Pork rinds

Eggs & Dairy:

3 one dozen egg cartons

5 packages stick butter

Package shredded mozzarella

Package shredded parmesan

2 packages block cream cheese

Container Greek yogurt

½ lb goat cheese

Other:

Package frozen strawberries

2 packages frozen raspberries

Jar sundried tomatoes

Jar green olives

Jar artichoke hearts

Container tahini paste

Bottle sesame oil

Cocoa butter

Bottle fish sauce

Cacao powder

Soy sauce

Recipe Index

Pork and Poultry 96

Beef and Lamb 101

Snacks and Sides 127

Printed in Great Britain
by Amazon